Dealing with Highly Anxious People

Dealing with Highly Anxious People

Smart Tactics to Cope with These People in Your Life

Nina W. Brown

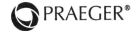 PRAEGER®

An Imprint of ABC-CLIO, LLC

Santa Barbara, California • Denver, Colorado

Library of Congress Cataloging-in-Publication Data

Names: Brown, Nina W., author.
Title: Dealing with highly anxious people : smart tactics to cope with these people in your life / Nina W. Brown.
Description: 1st Edition. | Santa Barbara : Praeger, 2019. | Includes bibliographical references and index. |
Identifiers: LCCN 2019025598 (print) | LCCN 2019025599 (ebook) | ISBN 9781440867651 (hardback) | ISBN 9781440867668 (ebook)
Subjects: LCSH: Anxiety. | Self-help techniques.
Classification: LCC BF575.A6 B76 2019 (print) | LCC BF575.A6 (ebook) | DDC 158.2—dc23
LC record available at https://lccn.loc.gov/2019025598
LC ebook record available at https://lccn.loc.gov/2019025599

ISBN: 978-1-4408-6765-1 (print)
        978-1-4408-6766-8 (ebook)

23 22 21 20 19   1 2 3 4 5

This book is also available as an eBook.

Praeger
An Imprint of ABC-CLIO, LLC

ABC-CLIO, LLC
147 Castilian Drive
Santa Barbara, California 93117
www.abc-clio.com

This book is printed on acid-free paper ∞

Manufactured in the United States of America

Contents

Preface

The idea for this book emerged from an experience I had with a very anxious person where I was frustrated because it seemed that there was always something that kept them in a state of anxiety. If one problem was solved, another one quickly took its place, and I had to hear about every one of them. In addition, I was trying to work with another person on a project and this person wasn't ever satisfied that I could do what was needed without them constantly checking on my progress, telling me what to do and how to do it, and just interrupting me with their concerns. I was always having to stop what I was doing to answer them about something that was not important, but they just had to have me available at that moment.

I described the idea of writing a book titled *Your Anxiety Is Driving Me Crazy*, to my daughter and to several colleagues, and every one of them said that they knew what I was talking about. My daughter, who teaches advanced courses in a high school, described some of her students who were extremely bright but were constantly anxious about almost everything and every day there was something new to be anxious about, so they looked to her for answers and relief. My colleagues described family members, friends, and other colleagues with whom they had similar experiences. It was at that point that I realized that many of us did not know how to understand this kind of anxiety, that it was different from the debilitating anxiety that needs medication and treatment, and that there were times when we did not want to see that person or hear about what was making them anxious. There did seem to be a need for understanding and coping with the common everyday variety of the overly anxiousness of some people, and so the book was developed.

What I am trying to do in the book is to characterize the worlds of the four identified categories of anxious people—the Worrier, the Complainer, the Micromanager, and the Nagger—their impact on you and others, and hope to provide you with some understanding of their anxiety. Also described are suggestions for how we play into their anxiousness by our need and desire to be helpful, how we tend to be open to "catching" their anxiousness and other feelings, and how we can respond and react more effectively for ourselves and for them.

Throughout the book you will find practical and easily implemented interventions, ideas for coping strategies and skills, and procedures for self-reflection and self-understanding. Presented are ways of understanding yourself and how your personality and other characteristics may be possible contributors to your personal reactions to the anxious person in your life. Central to what is presented is the assumption that you want to maintain the relationship because of its importance to you that there are limits for your responsibility for the other person's anxiety, and suggest strategies to guide you on how to develop helpful responses to their anxiety. It is my hope that you will be able to be more effective in interactions with the anxious person in your life and that your stress of dealing with others' anxiety will be reduced.

Acknowledgments

No book is written without input and help from others, and I want to thank the following people for their assistance with this project. Thanks are extended to Debbie Carvalko, the editor who helped guide the development of the book; to my daughter Linda Francis who gave me examples of how her adolescent high-achieving students were needlessly anxious about almost everything; and to my colleagues at the American Group Psychotherapy Society who presented on topics that shaped my thinking for the book.

CHAPTER ONE

Your Anxiety Is Driving Me Crazy!

It is the rare person who has not encountered a very anxious person, someone who is constantly anxious about even the smallest and most irrelevant thing. Do any of the following describe someone in your life?

- Frequently complains about almost everything and everyone
- Expects perfection and lets everyone know of this expectation
- Tells others what they should or ought to do
- Is excessively focused on details for others' tasks or work
- Is uncomfortable to work with on a project
- Insists that everything has to be "just so"
- Is usually very intense
- Cannot relax until they or others are "perfect," which never seems to happen
- Worries and fears negative outcomes for real and imagined future events
- Can readily imagine dire consequences and does so frequently
- Uses you as a sounding board for their worries and concerns
- Constantly sends you texts, e-mails, or phone calls about many concerns

Do you have someone in your life who is frequently anxious and looks to you for answers and reassurance to relieve their anxiety and their anxiety is driving you crazy at times? You want to help them, but it seems that there is always something that triggers their anxiety.

Anxiety as used here does not refer to someone who has received a formal diagnosis and is also receiving treatment for anxiety. As used here, the anxious person's state is not debilitating for them as would be for a diagnosed condition, but may be crazy-making for you and others because they never seem to stop dumping their thoughts and feelings on you, you cannot seem to give enough or provide satisfactory answers, and they never stop returning with their anxiety. More about their anxiety is discussed later.

This book is written for someone like you who has to live, work, and/or interact frequently with a very anxious person, and this presentation is intended to describe the anxious person's inner world(s), the impact of their behaviors and attitudes on you and on others, and to suggest ways to reduce or eliminate some of the negative impact on you. You want to be helpful and may even care deeply for them but may also have a deep desire that they would become less anxious about what seems to be just about everything. That possible deep desire is not addressed here because that is a wish for the other person to change. The focus here is on you and how you may be able to cope better.

The anxious person described here does not fit a diagnosis of anxiety as presented in *The Diagnostic and Statistical Manual of Mental Disorders* (*DSM*). Anxiety used here is descriptive of people who are Worriers, Micromanagers, Complainers, and Naggers.

Descriptors for Anxiety

A definition for anxiety discussed here has four descriptors, any or all of which may fit the person you have in mind as being anxious. The four components are worry in general, uneasiness about the future, ambiguous fear or dread, and persistent self-doubt.

Worry in general can be seen in the perceptions that the world is dangerous and that the person feels that they cannot survive unless they can prevent or overcome the danger. In addition, the person can worry about unknown dangers or just have a conviction that those exist. This ambiguity and apprehensions about dangers that are unknown, an inability to see or know what these are, as well as their apprehensions about their competencies to meet and conquer these dangers can produce considerable stress. These worries may not be real or logical or may not present in any order; they can be somewhat chaotic.

Uneasiness about the future can produce anxiety even if you are not a Worrier, and especially if you do try to stay current with local, regional, national, and international news and events. It is all too easy to get caught up in new stories and their extensions of interpretations and speculations that can then intensify any uneasiness. In addition, there are personal considerations that may produce uneasiness such as an illness, financial concerns, and employment.

Ambiguous fear or dread is just what it sounds like—nothing is happening or is anticipated to happen that produces anxiety and the person is unable to identify the source of their uneasiness, but the fear or dread is still there and exerting a negative influence. The state could be termed as existential anxiety, which can indicate that the anxiety is more about life in general—the human suffering, unfairness, and the universe's indifference—for which there are no definitive answers or solutions that, in turn, can produce even more anxiety.

Persistent self-doubt is both a source for anxiety and also a component for the other examples/definitions. This self-doubt can arise in response to being worried, having uneasiness about the future, and the ambiguous fear or dread about the capability or competency needed to meet and survive these unknown or known life challenges. While some of this is understandable and may be realistic, it can intensify the original anxiety and make it even more distressing.

The Worrier, Micromanager, Complainer, and Nagger can also have some of the following thoughts about themselves that add to their distress.

- "Woe is me" is an old lament about having troubles, trials, and tribulations as if others do not have similar events in their lives.
- "Things are awful, or will be" generalizes the anxiety to become central and devastating; they are unable to let go of the thought and may even intensify or exaggerate their anxiety.
- "It's up to me to fix it, or to prevent it" is a conviction that only that person can take care of it, and they don't know what to do.
- "I'll be blamed, seen as inadequate or stupid" for not having the power or control over the unspecified, unknown, and, maybe, the uncontrollable whatever.

These thoughts and feelings can be indicators of some grandiosity and omnipotence where the person has a belief or conviction that they should be able to see into the future, to prevent or to fix events that are not under their control or not their responsibility, or to take on tasks where no one person could be effective, and a whole host of other such thoughts.

Is There an Anxious Person in Your Life?

Let's stop and see if what is being discussed fits someone in your life that you term or could term as anxious. Think of someone you think could be anxious and complete the following scale about that person. This person may be a parent, a spouse or intimate partner, a close family member, a friend, a boss or supervisor, or a coworker.

Anxious Person Identification Scale

Directions: Get a sheet of paper and a writing instrument, find a place to work that is free from distractions and disruptions and that has a suitable surface for writing. Place a line of numbers from 1 to 30 down one side of the paper. Read each of the following descriptors, and place a checkmark beside the number if the person you are thinking about displays that behavior or attitude often or almost all of the time.

1. Complains about practically everything
2. Fusses over irrelevant details
3. Tries to manage how others do even minor tasks that they know how to do or could figure out how to do
4. Tries to ensure that every detail of just about everything must be exactly right
5. Expects others to act in accord with their demands, wishes, expectations, and the like
7. Readily highlights others' errors, mistakes, and the like
8. Closely watches others to see if they will make a mistake
9. Is reluctant to let others do things the way that they want to
10. Expects others to do things their way
11. Detail oriented about almost everything
12. Frets about what others may do, think, or say
13. Deeply desires that they do not make a mistake, which leads to dithering, procrastinating, and unnecessary delays
14. Verbalizes what others should or ought to do
15. Perceives others as inadequate or inferior when they make even minor mistakes
16. Readily verbalizes worries, complaints, and/or displeasure
17. Is unable to be pleased
18. Expects perfection especially from others
19. Seeks reassurance on a regular basis, for example, for being right
20. Intense when expressing thoughts, demands, wishes, reactions, and the like
21. Wonders out loud why others cannot seem to "get it right" and do what they want them to do, and other similar complaints

22. Becomes anxious about possible and/or improbable future events on a regular basis

23. Tends to be dramatic in actions and words

24. Seems to expect the worst to happen, as an outcome and of others

25. Panics easily

26. Cannot "see" or accept possible solutions when agitated

27. Is unable to screen out or manage intrusive and disruptive thoughts and feelings

28. Can be powerful emotional senders that contributes to others "catching" their feelings of distress

29. Collects mistakes others make and reminds them of those mistakes

30. Can fail to act for fear of being wrong, or of not being able to control outcomes

Scoring: Add up the checkmarks and use the following as a guide.

1–6 checkmarks: This person has few characteristics reflective of the anxious person.

7–12 checkmarks: The person has numerous characteristics, and these can be somewhat troubling.

13–19 checkmarks: The person has many characteristics, and many are troubling.

20+ checkmarks: The person has most of the characteristics, and these are very troubling.

Let's use the following as a guide for thinking about the anxious person in your life.

Checking 1–6 items on the scale suggests that the person may not be overly anxious much of the time, but still behaves and/or has attitudes that cause them to try and get rid of anxiety or moderate it by talking to you or others. The person has few of the descriptors and does not display them frequently so that these are less troubling to you or to the relationship.

Checking 7–12 items on the scale shows that the person has most of the described behaviors and attitudes and this suggests that they are anxious much of the time and can be seeking relief or answers from you and/or others. Encountering this person when they are anxious can be troubling when you have to interact with them on a regular basis.

If you checked 13–19 items on the scale about the anxious person in your life, you identified numerous behaviors and attitudes they display or have that can be troubling to you and to the relationship. This person can be in a state of anxiety very often and, because of the relationship, turn frequently to you for relief and answers even when there are no answers because of the ambiguous nature of the concern. The person has many of the descriptors that can be troubling to you, especially if you have to interact with them frequently or regularly, or are in a close relationship.

Checking over twenty items describe a person who is overly anxious much of the time and constantly seeks answers and relief. The person has all, or almost all, of the descriptors and displays these regularly and frequently, and these are very troubling to you.

Whatever the number of descriptors was for the person you identified, their anxiety can have a negative impact on you, and that may be impacting the quality of the relationship.

Some of Their Tendencies

Now that you have identified the level and extent to which the person you identified as being anxious exhibits their anxious behaviors, let's move to descriptors for some of their tendencies, behaviors, and attitudes that may be troubling to you, such as the following:

- Interrupts and disrupts you with unexpected phone calls, texts, e-mails, or in-person visits
- Seems to be hypersensitive to minor events, flaws, imperfections, and the like, and has a need to talk about these with you
- Frequently looks to you for solace, reassurance, and answers
- Often carps, kvetches, or fusses out loud when things are not to their liking, standards, or expectations
- Seems indifferent to the impact of their behavior on you and/or others
- Has unrealistic expectations of their self and of others
- Overly detail oriented for just about everything and may have an expectation that others act as they do
- Expects almost everyone to be sensitive and responsive to their concerns and to be so almost all of the time
- Tends to see problems and dangers where none exists
- Expects you to drop everything and attend to them
- Can lack insight or understanding of the source for their anxiety and/or perceive themselves as being realistic
- Is seldom empathic to your or others' concerns
- Does not hear, understand, or receive well suggestions about their anxiety or attempts to interject realism

These are only a few tendencies that may be troubling. It is probably more that they involve you frequently, consistently, and unexpectedly to listen to them and nothing you say or do seems to address their core concerns, and this can be troubling and crazy-making for you. You may even love and respect them and, at the same time, wish that they could find some other way to deal and cope with their constant anxiety. You want to be there for them in times of real need, but it seems that everything is perceived by them as a real need, and as important and urgent. Worse, it seems that they expect you to have their answers.

Four Categories

"Anxious" is a very nebulous word and not very descriptive for helping to understand the person or to suggest coping strategies that will help you, the person, and/or the relationship. What could be helpful is to try and describe four categories that can be descriptors for different kinds of anxious people. While each person is individualistic, unique, and special, putting them into general categories helps us describe some of their more troubling behaviors and attitudes and focuses suggestions for coping strategies you can use when interacting with them when they are anxious.

For the ease of discussion, four categories are presented: the Worrier, the Micromanager, the Complainer, and the Nagger. Each category begins with an illustrative vignette.

The Worrier

Selena was very worried. She woke up this morning with a headache and other pains. She was hoping that those would subside as she had a special presentation to make at her work, and she was also worried about that. In an effort to stop worrying about the presentation, she thought about her relationship with Jim and wondered where that was headed. From there, her thoughts went to her upcoming performance evaluation and her concern about receiving a fair evaluation, and from there, she started thinking about other incidents at work and with her family that were distressing.

In order to try to settle herself down for the presentation, she decided to call her best friend Cassie. When Cassie answered the phone, Selena blurted out that she was frantic because she had a headache, had a major presentation in an hour, and just knew she would not get a fair performance evaluation. She went on talking and scarcely let Cassie say a word. This behavior was not unusual for Selena; she typically called Cassie every time she was worried, sometimes call several times in a day. Few days went by without Cassie receiving at least one call from Selena. There were times when Cassie did not want to answer the phone or meet with Selena because Selena was almost always worried about something, and nothing Cassie said or did seemed to make a dent in her worries or continual worrying about things over which she had little or no control.

Following are some common behaviors and attitudes for many Worriers.

- Constantly stays alert in anticipation of future and/or possible vague dangers from all directions. They can be very imaginative about unrealistic possibilities.

- Usually perceives others as unable to care for themselves, or as not having the resources to adequately take care of themselves. They can constantly worry that it is their responsibility to take care of others who are capable of taking care of themselves.

- Feels that they should or must protect others from unknown dangers. Again, they do not recognize the limits of their responsibility for capable others.

- Expects the worse and does not appreciate it when the best happens, or when the worse does not happen. It's almost as if they revel in misfortunes, disasters, or troubles. Worse is that they cannot appreciate good fortune or outcomes.

- Dithers in decision making or problem solving. They are so worried about possibilities and imaginary disaster that they cannot think clearly enough to create or see solutions or alternatives or to make decisions. Worse for some is that they do make a decision and then worry about that decision in every way possible.

When they worry they make many associations and that extends their concerns to many things that are not under their control. Their thoughts can hop from topic to topic.

The Micromanager

The members of Brad's team were very productive, but many of those members were irritated that Brad checked up on their work and progress so frequently. While his expertise was helpful at times, it also seemed that he did not have confidence in them to do their assignments or to do them well. He checked with each person on the team several times a day, either by phone, e-mail, or appearing in person. He wanted to know in detail what they were doing, and why, and how they were doing whatever it was. Some team members liked to talk about what they were doing, while others wanted to be left alone to do their work.

Brad's micromanaging was also evidenced at home for such tasks as loading the dishwasher. He demanded that the dishwasher be loaded a particular way and checked to ensure that it was done the way that he wanted. He also insisted that other family members attend to other household tasks with the detail that he wanted.

It should be noted that the Micromanager does not limit their tactics to any one area of their lives where others are concerned. If someone is a Micromanager in one setting, they tend to be the same in all of their other settings. Following are some common actions, beliefs, and attitudes that characterize the Micromanager.

- Does not trust others' competencies, abilities, or their sense of responsibility.
- Extremely detail oriented, mainly noticing flaws, imperfections, and mistakes.
- Wants everything done in accord with their exacting standards even when their vision of the standards have not been communicated.
- Expects others to report and relate in detail what they propose to do and what they did, and to provide rationales for each of these. Some Micromanagers can even expect others to do this on a regular basis without being told to do so.
- Checks in with others often. A Micromanager can be intrusive and disruptive because their anxiety compels them to constantly monitor others by checking in with them. Micromanagers can delude themselves sometimes that they are being helpful and that others appreciate their attention. However, the constant checking in interferes with others' thoughts and attention to the task at hand.
- Constantly questions others about their actions, intents, thoughts, and the like. They may perceive this as welcomed interest and attention, but most likely the constant questions are neither welcomed nor appreciated much of the time.
- Expects to be blamed if others make mistakes or when everything is not perfect. It is interesting that this is their expectation because it is likely that they blame others when things don't go right or as planned.

The Micromanager is concerned about how they are perceived when they have to rely on others whom they do not believe can be trusted on their own. One key to managing a Micromanager is to try and keep them apprised of what is done, what is proposed to be done, and how you intend to do it. This may not be consistent with how you like to work, but it can keep the intrusions less.

The Complainer (Carp, Kvetch, Fuss, Fret)

Felix wished that other people would pay attention to what they did or were supposed to do as much as he did. He fretted about their seemingly inability or indifference to doing what they "ought" to do or to do so to his satisfaction. He also felt that it was his duty to call their and everyone's attention to what he considered as their mistakes, deficit, and other errors. Nothing was too minor to escape his attention. For example, at the last family dinner when others were praising the roast, Felix said that the roast was too dry and had not been cooked at the correct temperature. He also complained that the other dishes were not to his liking, or "as they should be."

His tendency to complain about almost everything and everyone, and to do so constantly, had been called to his attention, but he did not feel that those charges had any validity. He felt that he was doing only what needed to be done and that others should do as he did as that was the right thing to do. There always seemed to be something for him to single out for a complaint.

The Complainer can have the following behaviors, beliefs, and attitudes.

- Their discomfort or distress or perception of what "should" be is their priority. If they don't like what is happening, then it's because someone else did not do what they should or were supposed to do to prevent the Complainer from the discomfort.

- They desire that others recognize and admire their fortitude and suffering. They are quick to voice their suffering, point out how they have to endure this and other things, and can even say that they should be admired for putting up with everything that isn't right.

- Nothing ever seem good enough or satisfactory. They can always, or almost always, find fault with anything or anyone. There is always something that doesn't meet their (unspecified) standards.

- They suck the pleasure out of just about everything. Having to hear complaints is not pleasurable, especially when these are constant, about trivia, may not matter or affect someone negatively, and reduce enjoyment of everything else. It would be acceptable for them to have the complaint(s) if they didn't feel that they had to verbalize them to you.

- They are very discontented with their selves and with others. Seeking perfection for everything and everyone is futile and exhausting. Nothing or almost nothing is satisfying and up to their expectations, and they feel that they always fall short by not being able to compel others to do what they want even when they haven't let this be known. This produces deep disappointment for them and about others.

- When help or advice is extended, it is often rejected as not being possible, or that it will not work, or that it doesn't seem right for their circumstances. They seem to have an internal vision of what is right that they assume is also the vision that others have, so that offers to help, or to fix it, are rejected by them because what others are proposing does not meet their internal vision, which remains hidden and unspecified.

- They appear to go out of their way to ensure that others know of their displeasure and how things are not right or as they "should" be. They do not suffer in silence or, if they don't speak out at first, somewhere along the line they make their displeasure known, usually to you. While you may not have any responsibility for what produces their complaint, this does not prevent them from letting you in on their disappointment, displeasure, and discontent. Some Complainers can even let their discontent be known in public to and about others.

You may have to accept that neither you nor anyone else is going to be able to make the complaining cease. There are things you can do in the moment to manage your and their feelings, but that is only for the moment and when they get a chance, more complaints will emerge. Your understanding of the Complainer and judicious use of coping strategies are critical to your well-being.

The Nagger

Sue did not relish having to remind her family, friends, or coworkers of what they promised, needed to do, or should change so as to become better. However, it seemed to her that without her reminders, other people would not follow through or would continue to make the same mistakes, or something dire would happen that could be avoided. She felt that she spent most of her time keeping others on the right track, and, if she did not remind them frequently enough, they would forget.

Sue was also very demanding in other ways, such as expecting others to not object to her interruptions or to remind them of what she thought that they should or ought to do. She also thought that they should be grateful that she remembered what they were supposed or needed to do or that others should attend to doing what she wanted them to do. Sometimes, others just wished that she would shut up.

Some characteristic behavior and attitudes are as follows:

- Talks a lot, especially when providing reminders to others. They are quick to remind you to do something over and over again, provide reasons why you should do what they say, and talk about the times when you failed to do something. They never seem to forget anything you did or failed to do that led to a negative or uncomfortable outcome.

- Believes that others will not do what they are expected or supposed to do unless they receive many reminders. Naggers seem to have an expectation that others are just waiting to goof off and be trifling, and should immediately do what they are told to do, or will never remember unless they are reminded several times. They want things to be done immediately even when what they are nagging about is in the future and not possible at the time.

- Expects others to remember details, to become distracted, and/or to ignore or forget their responsibilities. Part of what seems to fuel the nagging is their belief that others will not know or remember what needs to be done, and it is up to them to stay on top of everything or nothing will get done. Even when this belief is seldom or never valid, it still exerts its influence on the Nagger.

- Nothing is done quickly enough. It doesn't help the relationship that the Nagger can expect quick and prompt compliance even if there are other more immediate and important things to be done. It can seem that others can never comply quickly enough for them. It's almost as if the Nagger expects their dictates to be completed on the spot and with no time lag.

- Perceives their constant reminders as being helpful to others, in spite of evidence to the contrary. Some Naggers may notice the negative impact of their nagging on others and dismiss their reactions as not being important. Or, the other person sometimes gives in just to cease their nagging and complies, but that compliance just reinforces the Nagger's belief that they are correct to give these constant reminders. Some truly believe that they are merely being helpful.

There are times when the Nagger's reminders are helpful, and you may want to remember this when you have negative reactions to their nagging.

Similarities and Positives among Categories

The previous section provided some descriptors for differentiating between the categories, and there may also be additional identifiers. These anxious people do tend to be alike in some ways. The main reason for the different categories is so that the proposed coping strategies and skills presented in later chapters can be adapted to better fit the anxious person in your life. The similarities may be helpful for you to try and understand something about their inner worlds and experiencing. Understanding can allow you to have more patience with them at times, prevent some of your frustration, and encourage you to develop personalized strategies.

The inner world of anxious people can be filled with thoughts, feelings, and ideas about their adequacy, their competencies and abilities, self-blame, and unrealistic expectations of their selves. Some of these can be associated with earlier experiences, unresolved issues, and/or unfinished business. But I am not trying to find causes or to assign blame. Rather, the focus and intent here is on trying to understand what may be triggering or fueling their anxiety, thus impelling them to try to reduce their distressing thoughts and feelings through their interactions with you.

A central thought to keep in mind is that they do not see or appreciate the extent of the impact that their anxiety has on you.

At some level, they question their self-adequacy and may even feel inadequate, which is not unlike what many other people do and feel. For example, it would not be unusual to ask yourself at times, "Am I up to this?," or "Can I do this?." However, the difference between you and the anxious person can be that they deeply and persistently question their self-adequacy and never really feel adequate, thus need constant reassurance.

Some basic similarities are as follows:

- Talking with someone seems to provide momentary relief.
- This relief cannot be maintained; something else emerges that is distressing, and so they continue to unload on others.
- They can have a strong need or desire for perfection for almost everything.
- As a group they seem to be unable to distinguish between what is under their control and what is not, or they seem to be able to accept their limitation.
- Many can be deeply insecure but mask this with grandiose thoughts and feelings.
- Many are unable to engage in flexible thinking.

Most of the characteristics seem to be negative, but there are also other characteristics that are positive.

1. Some Worriers and Micromanagers can often anticipate some problems, and this allows for actions to prevent or reduce the negative impact of these problems. Anticipating possible glitches or other barriers can suggest interventions that can be helpful. For example, anticipating needs and actions for a possible natural disaster allows for preparation such as gathering of food and water in the event of a power outage.

2. They can adhere to a personal code of values or conduct. Their rigid thinking and persistence in "doing the right thing" can help reduce errors and increase positive outcomes. For example, following directions, obeying rules and laws, or abiding by established procedures for the job or profession can provide for quick interventions when there are unanticipated problems that arise and can also promote positive outcomes.

3. There is a saying that "the devil is in the details," and the person who can visualize what those details are can anticipate what is needed to ensure satisfactory results and outcomes. There are careers and occupations that call for this kind of attention to details, such as event planners, renovators, proofreaders, political strategists, copyeditors, and party planners. Their tendency to be detail oriented can assist to achieve satisfactory results.

4. The anxiety can be energizing for them although it is exhausting to others. They expend considerable energy in thinking about possibilities, checking with and on others, revisiting things to ensure that every detail is accounted for, and other such actions. Relaxing is difficult, and they want to ensure perfection and that requires energy.

5. They are not always wrong. Although their actions can be irritating at times, they can be correct: for example, the Worrier who predicts about an improbable event that does happen, such as a company being sold that results in job losses; the Micromanager who finds out that an important point was not addressed for a costly project proposal; the Complainer who points out that an oil spill on a floor was not cleaned properly and is dangerous; and the Nagger whose constant reminders ensured that critical documents were available when needed for the IRS tax review.

Your Roles and the Relationship

Much of what has been presented does not take into account the roles or relationship you have with the anxious person in your life. Knowing and understanding your role will help you find or create the appropriate response to be consistent with the relationship. For example, your role as a friend will necessitate a different response or coping strategy than your role as a boss or co-worker, or as a spouse/partner, or as an adult child. In addition, your role contributes to your perceptions and reactions, interacts with your personality, and is influenced by conscious and unconscious cultural assumptions and expectations you may have about how to relate and behave. Adding to this is that the role you play can differ with the relationship you have with the anxious person in your life and with the situation.

Some basic assumptions can guide you in learning to understand your anxious person, how to better manage your feelings and reactions, and can suggest more constructive responses. The basic assumptions that you may wish to select are as follows:

- You want to preserve and enhance the relationship. You do not want to do anything that will destroy the relationship or have a negative effect on it.
- Adopt the perspective that The Worrier, Micromanager, Complainer, or Nagger is unlikely to change. Yes, they can change, but only if they want to but they probably do not see any reason to change and nothing you can do or say will cause them to change. It is very helpful for you to accept this although it may be unpalatable.
- Ensure that your responses always use courtesy, tact, and civility. It is essential that you not show your exasperation, anger, or similar reactions because that will not help them or the relationship.

- You can experience some distress that lingers after interactions with the anxious person until you learn some emotional insulation and work to reduce your emotional susceptibility.
- Common feelings you may experience are frustration, irritation, helplessness, dread and apprehension, caring and concern for their welfare, inadequacy to resolve or please, and/or a desire to get away.

What Is Next

Chapter 1 presented an overview of the anxious person described in this book, suggested ways to identify an anxious person in your life, proposed four categories, and presented some characteristics, both positive and negative. Chapter 2 describes some possible impacts on you when that person becomes anxious and presents some forces that may cause you to be open to their anxiety such as emotional susceptibility and your psychological boundary strength. Chapter 3 starts the process for presenting strategies and skills that can be helpful when interacting with the anxious person. This chapter focuses on immediacy, that is, when you are not anticipating them presenting you with their current anxiety-provoking thoughts and feelings. Chapter 4 continues this presentation with the focus on long-term suggestions and strategies. Chapter 5 is intended to show you how to better defend yourself and prevent frustration as well as better understand the limits of your personal responsibilities for others who can take care of themselves and how to assess the severity of the perceived threat to them. Chapter 6 seeks to describe the anxious person's blind spots, why they cannot see solutions or are indifferent to the impact of their anxiety on you and on others, and why it is futile to try to change them. Chapter 7 continues this description with a focus on their irrational and chaotic inner world that leads them to experience and convey their anxiety. Chapters 8 and 9 present strategies for the four categories that takes into account your relationship with that person. These chapters present specific suggestions for understanding and responses when the anxious person is a parent, a spouse or intimate partner, a friend, a boss, or a coworker. The final chapter focuses on you and how you can identify and address your unproductive anxiety although yours is not as intense as any of those in the four categories.

CHAPTER TWO

Why and How You Are Affected by Their Anxiety

The anxious person you identified in Chapter 1 turns to you to vent, relieve their anxiety in some way, to advise them what to do to feel better, and/or to fix whatever is causing them this anxiety. The positive side is that they usually feel better after talking with you, having received some of what they were looking for. On the other hand, you usually feel worse than you felt before interacting with them. This chapter discusses how some of your personal characteristics act to produce your discomfort during and after they unload their concerns and some actions that can help reduce their negative impact on you. Among the topics that are presented are emotional contagion, psychological boundaries, emotional susceptibility, the extent of your personal responsibility, your external and internal needs and their roles, descriptions for how they suck you into their anxieties through their projections and your projective identification, and how your personal growth and development can help both of you.

Emotional Contagion

Some people are powerful projectors of emotions, and it can be very difficult to block the emotions they project, even when you are not in a relationship where you have psychological investment in that person. For example, actors earn their living by projecting emotions to audience. You have no connection with them, they are playing their roles, and you can still end up feeling the projected emotion. Children are also powerful projectors.

The younger they are, the more powerful their projections can seem. If you are not shielded, you can easily feel the emotions that infants project.

The projectors in your life, however, who are cause for concern, are neither actors nor children. These are senders who project their distressing feelings; you catch these and become distressed. These senders are using their feelings to manipulate you into doing what they want you to do. Remember, for both of you, this manipulation takes place on the unconscious level. You are not consciously aware of the sender's projections, and that person is not aware that he or she is projecting.

The more primitive emotions of fear and anger also tend to be the most powerful ones, and you are probably reacting to these most of the time. To illustrate, suppose you are with someone who is a powerful projector, and that person wants you to do something, but is not sure you will cooperate. This person can unconsciously think that they (1) are entitled to get what is wanted; (2) has a right to expect and/or manipulate you to give what is wanted; and (3) they are *fearful* of not getting the need met.

What can happen in this case is that the sender's fear is projected onto you, and the sender then reacts to you as if you were fearful, for example, moving closer, using a soothing voice, and caressing or patting you to reassure you that you need not be frightened. You react to the fear by accepting the unwanted soothing thus addressing the projected fear as if it was your fear. If the sender can soothe you then they are not fearful, but you continue to carry the fear and may become very afraid.

Your reaction and feelings are much more intense if you identify with any or all of the projected fear. You incorporate that fear, make it part of yourself, and then become manipulated by it. This is another example of projective identification. Your psychological and physical boundaries have been violated, and you are not consciously aware of the intrusion.

Your Vulnerability

Other people can sense your vulnerability. Unknowingly you may send out signals that indicate you are available for manipulation and exploitation. I know that seems like harsh statement, but it is important for you to increase your awareness of how you may contribute to some of your own distress. Your insecurity; lack of confidence; spongy, brittle, or soft psychological boundaries; your need for connections and reassurance; and your desire to be loved and valued put you in apposition where others can sense that you are open to manipulation and exploitations. Add this to your conscious desires to be a caring, thoughtful, considerate, and sensitive person. Such desires are commendable but not helpful in your present circumstances.

Your Emotional Susceptibility

Before continuing, it may be helpful to get some objective measure of your own susceptibility. The following questions describe some behaviors and attitudes that suggest sensitivity to others' feelings, which may result in considerable personal cost to you, or in self-destructive behavior. As you read each question, ask yourself how often this fits you.

Evidence of Emotional Susceptibility Scale

1. Doing something you do not want to do, just to please another person?
2. Wishing you had not let someone persuade you to do something that you felt was imprudent or wrong?
3. Wondering how you got into an uncomfortable situation?
4. Feeling like a fool for having trusted someone who betrayed you?
5. Giving of yourself to someone, only to find that the person did not value you as you did them?
6. Surprised at the feeling, or intensity of feeling, you have in an interaction with another person?
7. Feeling beaten down by accusations that you act selfishly and that you are self-centered?
8. Becoming guilty or ashamed when someone tells you that you don't care for them, because if you did, you would do what that person wants you to do?
9. Giving someone sympathy because they are sad, but then becoming and staying sad yourself?
10. Interacting with someone who is angry and frustrated, and when it's time to leave, you find yourself in an emotional tailspin, when you were okay before the interaction took place?
11. Working hard to ensure harmony and feeling guilty and responsible when there is conflict?

At this point, the causes of your susceptibility will not be addressed. The intent here is on establishing what you may be doing, thinking, and/or feeling that leads to you "catching" others' emotions, and the degree of distress your emotional susceptibility causes you.

If you found that many (8+) items fit you, then you may experience frequent distress due to your inability to resist catching others' emotions and/or feeling that you must please them. There are times when you find yourself acting in a way that is inconsistent with your intentions, values, morals, or self-interest. The residual feelings stay with you for a long time, and you may berate yourself, feel guilty or ashamed, and make vows to change only to find yourself again in the same or a similar situation a short time later.

If you found that five or more of the items fit you, then you may tend to find yourself in situations where their emotions are triggered by others, suggesting that you have a lot of emotional susceptibility. You may even realize what is happening at the time, but you feel helpless to stop it or to prevent it from happening again. You may even chide yourself and make plans for how to prevent it in the future, and on occasion, you are able to control your emotional susceptibility. However, all too often, it still happens, and you are distressed at your inability to adequately shield yourself from others' emotions.

If you had fewer than five of the items that seem to fit, you may experience catching others' emotions infrequently but you may still be troubled when you do catch these. You probably have the needed elements in your character to shield yourself emotionally but are unable to employ them in certain situations. Your susceptibility is limited and focused.

Psychological Boundaries

Psychological boundaries are the most difficult to describe as they are internal and unique to the individual. Your psychological boundary strength is also related to the extent to which you have achieved psychological separation and individuation (self-identity) from your parent or primary caretaker. Psychological boundaries are those that define the "self," that is, a deep understanding of where you end and an equally deep understanding of other people as distinct, different individuals. Those who do not have this understanding perceive others as extensions of self, and thus under their control, so that they can order, manipulate, and use others in the service of their self.

Psychological boundary strength also contributes to the capacity to be empathic. Empathy is experienced when you voluntarily open the boundaries around your essential inner self to be able to experience what the other person is feeling without losing the sense of your self as being separate and distinct from the other person. You do not "catch" the other person's feelings inadvertently, or become enmeshed with their feelings, or become overwhelmed with the intensity of their feelings, or become manipulated to unconsciously accept and act on the other person's feelings. You can end the empathic attunement at any time and not carry lingering aspects of the other person's feelings when you have sufficient psychological boundary strength.

Strong psychological boundaries can be seen in one's ability to:

- Be appropriately assertive
- Say "no" and stick to it
- Express wishes and desires openly and appropriately
- Respect others' boundaries
- Be appropriately empathic
- Give and receive favors
- Form and maintain satisfying relationships free of exploitation

Building and developing resilient and stronger psychological boundaries will enable you to withstand the intrusion and assaults from others that lead to violations of your boundaries as well as resisting projective identifications.

Types of Boundaries

Four categories of psychological boundaries are presented: resilient, soft, inflexible, and spongy. Read these to get a better idea of the strength of your psychological boundaries and determine if they are sufficiently strong,

Resilient boundaries allow you to adapt to different situations where you can have a strong or rigid boundary when necessary that does not allow your "self" be violated or intruded upon, to resist and repel projections and projective identifications. However, but, when appropriate, you can be flexible and open so that you can allow yourself to feel empathy for another person. Resilient boundaries permit you to choose when to be closed off and when to be open.

Soft boundaries allow you to easily become enmeshed or overwhelmed by others' feelings or demands. The lack of strength for your psychological boundaries permits others to manipulate or bully you into doing something you do not want to do. These boundaries are fragile and cannot adequately protect the essential inner self. People with soft boundaries cannot choose to be empathic as they are more likely to become enmeshed or overwhelmed.

Inflexible boundaries are unyielding and rigid to protect the self, and are also the armor that prevents you from experiencing empathy or connecting to others in meaningful ways. Such boundaries serve to keep the person isolated, alienated, and unable to make satisfying emotional connections with others since the person is more preoccupied with keeping the self safe.

Spongy boundaries are those that have some strength and can repel some projections and projective identifications. However, these boundaries are also capable of becoming penetrated, usually without the owner's knowledge or permission, and this allows the person to be unduly influenced, manipulated, and controlled by others. Although it is possible to be open in some areas to allow some empathy to be experienced, spongy boundaries can be so impenetrable that large parts of the self are closed to being open enough to experience empathy.

Personal Responsibility

Some emotional susceptibility can be triggered by your conscious and unconscious internal perceptions, assumptions about yourself and about others, and other irrational and unrealistic expectations. These internal states may have been incorporated into your essential inner self from your parents and other significant people in your early life; some were developed from interactions with others including the immediate community's culture, and others are how you internalized and made sense of your experiences. Your choices of what to internalize as parts of your essential inner self have roles for how you see yourself today, your self-adequacy, self-competency, and self-efficacy. They also play a role in how you are reacting to the anxious person in your life. Read the following list and notice the ones that fit you as you are today.

Contributing Perceptions, Thoughts, and Assumptions

1. I am responsible for how others feel, meaning that I should work to ensure that they have positive feelings.
2. If there is disharmony, I am at fault because I did not prevent it, and I need to work to fix what caused the disharmony.
3. I must never do or say anything that could upset another person because how they feel is my responsibility.
4. If I do not prevent or engage in any conflict, that means I will be abandoned or destroyed.
5. When someone makes me feel good, that means that person likes me and liking is necessary for my survival.
6. When someone likes me, that means they will take care of me, and that person has my best interests at heart.
7. I feel many times that I need to do things I do not want to do so others will be happy and approve of me.
8. It is always selfish to put my needs before others' needs.
9. If I am agreeable, everyone will like and approve of me.

10. People will like me if I always say pleasant things.
11. I need to take care of others so that they will like me.
12. If I love someone enough, they will love me in return.
13. I feel worthwhile only if I have someone to love me.
14. I only feel alive and excited when I'm with the person I love.

Did you find many or a few of the statements that are reflective of how you think and feel? Let's examine each of these to better understand how they can contribute to your emotional vulnerability and susceptibility and how they are not rational or logical.

Other People's Feelings

Taking responsibility for others' feelings puts you in a place where you work hard to ensure that others have positive feelings even if you end up doing something you don't want to do, or is not in your best interests to do just to ensure that the other person has only positive feelings. However, just as others are not responsible for your feelings, you are not responsible for the feelings that others experience. You cannot cause others to have a particular feeling; they choose to have the feeling, or they identified with all or part of a projection and are now acting on it. Either way, their feelings are their responsibility, not yours.

You may have incorporated the notion or conviction that you are responsible for other people's feelings early in your life through one or both parents' expectations that you were to be responsible for their emotional well-being. Or, you may be acting on a learned assumption that holds you responsible for how other people feel.

No matter what your reason for holding this belief might be, it is a *faulty* assumption and it contributes to your emotional susceptibility. For example, others such as the anxious person in your life, a relative, a boss, or a parent, may manipulate you by:

- Asking you, "Don't you want to make me feel good?"
- Telling you that you caused them to feel a particular feeling
- Criticizing you for not paying enough attention to their feelings
- Expecting you to take care of them, and saying so on numerous occasions

It is not easy to overcome this notion of being responsible for others' feelings, especially if the notion has been ingrained from childhood experiences and may not be conscious on your part.

Ensure Harmony

You may believe that you are the person who has a responsibility to ensure that there is always harmony, and, if disharmony exists, you must deal with it, make it go away, and restore harmony to the situation. You can stay on edge and anxious to be alert for hints or signals of disharmony, so that you can spring into action.

Although harmony is desirable, always having to maintain harmony works against your best interests and your well-being. You can be manipulated by others who will use your desire for harmony and your good nature to get you to do what they want you to do and you may go along with whatever is it they want just to be agreeable or to keep the peace.

For example, you may have a parent who wants you to do their errands for them, even though the parent can easily do them. The fact that you are inconvenienced is of no concern to the parent. But you don't want to say "no" because that would upset the parent, and you feel that you must preserve harmony at all costs. The intensity of the need you have for harmony, and the assumption that you are responsible for maintaining it, can leave you at the mercy of other people's wishes and needs.

No one person is responsible for maintaining harmony. Everyone bears some responsibility for situations to be harmonious, and it is a bit grandiose to expect that you are sufficiently powerful to ensure that harmony will always prevail. There are limits to your responsibility and for what you can control.

Upsetting Others

How do you feel when someone gets upset about something you said? Do you rush to explain, change what you meant, or try to soothe that person? Do you tend to be tentative and careful in what you say to others for fear of upsetting them, and then rationalize your carefulness with the thought that you are just being sensitive? If you answered yes to any or all of the questions, then you are using assumptions that are faulty. Some other conscious or unconscious thoughts you can have when another person becomes upset are the following:

- If I said something to upset them, then they will not like me.
- What I said caused them to think that I'm insensitive.
- I feel guilty because I did something wrong or otherwise they would not be upset.
- I should not have said what I did because it made them upset.

- It upsets me when I say or do something that (seems to cause) causes someone to be upset.
- How could I do something so stupid?

All these thoughts are focused on you and your feelings. In one sense, you are taking responsibility for your feelings, but you are also blaming yourself and taking responsibility for what the other person is feeling.

If, or when, something you say triggers another person's feelings, that's all it is—a trigger. Their feelings are triggered because of *their* issues, unfinished business, current emotional state, and so forth. The other person could choose to not become upset, or to work on their underlying issues so that their feelings are not triggered, or choose to do other personal growth and development work.

Having to stay alert all the time to ensure that you aren't on the verge of saying something that might upset someone else is emotionally draining, and can translate into physical tension. It is also futile because there is always someone to get upset about something. Taking that stance also means that you must be alert to any nonverbal cues of distress that others display, and, as you will see later, that can open you up to being emotionally manipulated.

Preventing Conflict

Conflicts can range in intensity from mild disagreements about something of little or no consequence to fierce battles. The most common perception about conflict deems it bad, undesirable, attacking, and destructive. If this is your definition of conflict, then you probably do everything in your power to avoid it. You may even give in, do what someone else wants you to do, or act against your values and principles in order to avoid engaging in conflict with having to say no or assert yourself in other ways.

Conflict, when managed well, can be constructive and help to strengthen relationships. Disagreements can be a way to clarify values and opinions, reveal beliefs and attitudes, and understand what is significant and important for each other. Conflicts do not have to be win-lose situations; each person can win. You do not have to give in to the other person, nor they to you. When you are so afraid of losing the relationship if you were to disagree with the other person, you do not have a strong relationship; moreover you may be opening yourself up to being manipulated by the other person.

Conflict is not always unavoidable. If you choose to avoid conflict with another person, you may end up with internal conflict. Furthermore, your avoidance may be misinterpreted by the other person, leading them to believe that you can be manipulated to do whatever that person wants, and the person will be correct in that assessment. Your faulty assumption about conflict can put you in this position.

Fear of Abandonment or Destruction

The two basic fears we all have to differing degrees are the fear of being abandoned and the fear of being destroyed. These fears appear to be present from birth, some remain on the unconscious level, but whether conscious or unconscious they can be components in the relationships we form. That is, we are attracted to others with the expectations that they will neither abandon nor destroy us.

These fears can be triggered easily when you have not fortified your "self" to have confidence that you can survive independently from another person. When you have a fortified self, you understand what loneliness is, and you can make constructive use of it rather than becoming anxious and forming unproductive and unsatisfying relationships to avoid feeling lonely.

Your openness to catching another's emotions can cause your fears to become triggered or lead you to incorporate and act on the other person's projective identifications which could be their fears about abandonment or destruction and that would intensify your fears and could, at the same time, cause you to act on the sender's fears.

If the other person fears either abandonment or destruction, and you catch and identify with those fears, you will act to prevent those fears, which were their fears and are now your fears, from being realized. This is what the other person will have wanted or intended in the first place, but now you are distressed and fearful and the other person is not because their fears were offloaded onto you. Sufficient psychological boundary strength can prevent you from catching, identifying, and acting on the sender's (such as the anxious person in your life) feelings.

Feeling Good and Being Liked

The desire to be liked is a usual human desire. However, when there is a deep-seated need to be liked that is extended to all relationships or to even most relationships, that need can then be sensed by others and used by them to manipulate, seduce, coerce, and bully you. You may be willing to go along with what another person proposes simply because they make you feel valued, important, and good. Your need and belief might lead you astray because you are more focused on getting this need met than you are on what that person is asking or demanding that you do for their benefit.

Of course, it is possible—even likely—that others do care for you and they do want you to feel good. You may have friends, lovers, and family members who meet this description, and when true, they can provide valuable emotional support. There is also the very real possibility that some of the people whom you think care for you are using your need to be liked and feel good to meet their needs. Yes, they will like you so long as they can manipulate you to meet their needs, but that is not in your best interest.

You will want to examine your need to be liked, the extent to which you compromise your values, and so forth, to please another person so that they will continue to like you. You will also want to examine the psychological and emotional costs you pay for continuing to hold and act on your need.

Your Best Interests

You likely believe that you are a caring person in other aspects of your life since you care for the welfare of the anxious person in your life, but this can be misleading and lead you to believe that others are also caring people and that they have your best interests at heart. Examine the following beliefs to determine if they are working for you:

- The belief that liking equates with caring. You may want to examine this belief to determine its validity or how it may be contributing to your distress.
- The unrealistic belief that others have a responsibility to take care of you just as you may be taking care of them.
- The belief that you need someone to take care of you or you will not survive.
- The belief that the other person (such as the anxious person in your life) is not independent and capable of taking care of themselves.

You may live by a belief such as the following: when you like someone, you do what you can to take care of that person with the hope and expectation that your caring will be reciprocated. Over time, you may have modified that belief in the face of your experiences that this was not true, and you may have had many disappointments. But your disappointments may not have deterred you and you continue to give of yourself and received little or no caring in return.

It is wonderful to be in a relationship with someone who does have your best interests at heart, someone you can trust not to hurt you, someone who does their best to take care of you. This is the basis for a deep, meaningful, and satisfying relationship. It's both an ideal and a realistic possibility and a goal worth pursuing. It is also a complement to you that you are willing to give to the anxious person in your life. You may not be getting the same considerations from the anxious person in your life.

Trust—Misplaced or Realistic?

Not trusting anyone to have your best interests at heart is not a desirable condition. You want to strike a reasonable balance between not trusting anyone and trusting everyone. Also, you will need to gain a clearer understanding of what constitutes reasonable limits on your expectations of others, even those who like you. Yes, you should be able to trust your family, friends, and other loved ones, but there are also limits as to what you should expect from them.

Then, too, there are those who are friendly and/or appear to be loving, but, in reality, they use others to meet their personal needs. It is a mistake to expect such people to have your interest as one of their priorities. What will be helpful for you is to be open to the best interpretations that others do like you and will care for you, but it is also helpful that you understand that their caring has limits. You can help yourself by being willing to take care of yourself and to not make demands or place unrealistic expectation on others.

Wanting Others' Approval

Wanting the approval of others can be one of the most self-destructive and dangerous needs that you can have as this can cause you to feel considerable guilt and shame when someone doesn't seem to approve of you. This need is very destructive when someone wants you to do something you do not want to do or that is not in your best interests, and you comply just to get or keep their approval. It does not matter if the other person is a family member, friend, boss, or lover.

Constantly trying to win someone's approval can be destructive because doing so

- gives power and control over you to that person,
- can cause you to violate your personal standards and integrity,
- ignores your personal values, morals, and beliefs that you live by,
- promotes your compliance with being manipulated, and
- encourages you to act inconsistent with your best interests.

However, you will still want to consider carefully what others want you to do and evaluate the validity of the claims on your time and attention. For example, if your parent wants you to visit a sick friend or relative, you may want to honor their request. What is important is this: *No matter what someone else wants you to do, your motivation should not be to make that person like you or to have them approve of you.* If you do what is requested, do it because you want to do it, not to be liked.

When you have the opportunity, you may want to reflect on why your need to be liked and approve of by everyone or almost everyone is so strong. You may want to analyze why being liked is so important to you that you are willing to compromise significant parts of yourself, such as your values, to satisfy this need. You may also want to think deeply about your current and past relationships and identify when and how often your need to be liked resulted in you being persuaded to act in a way that caused you distress just to please the other person.

Self-care

There is a vast difference between taking care of yourself appropriately and self-absorption. The first is a healthy response, and the second reflects selfishness and underdeveloped narcissism. It is not selfish to put your needs ahead of satisfying another's needs or desires *some of the time.* However, giving your needs top priority all of the time reflects a constant self-absorption that can impair your relationships. Nonetheless, always giving others' needs priority over your own implies that you consider yourself less important than others, and this attitude can promote emotional susceptibility.

It is, however, difficult to define or describe the phrase "some of the time" in this context. One reason for the difficulty is that even when you may think that you are putting another's needs first, you may be acting from your deep-seated need to be liked, not because of the other person's need or manipulation of you. In any case, there are definitely times when it is in your best interest to put your own needs first, but these times depend on the circumstances, the others involved, your relationships with them, and many other variables. Always putting others' needs ahead of your own can lead to your manipulation by others. They learn how to trigger your guilt and shame by calling you selfish even when you are not being selfish.

If you hold the belief that it is selfish to put your needs ahead of satisfying others' wishes, then you are not taking good care of yourself. You can learn how to balance self-interest and the appropriate nurturing of others. Your priorities shift and change depending on the situations and the relationship with the other person and what their needs are at the time, but it is healthier for you to be able to give yourself priority when appropriate.

Being Agreeable

It is true that some people will like you if you are agreeable, but it is also true that some people will consider your agreeableness as an invitation to take advantage of you. Others may consider it merely superficial, and still others will wonder why you do not assert yourself more often. You may believe that you must be agreeable for others to like you and that liking you is essential for your survival. One difficulty is that the achievement of such amiability causes you to ignore or conceal your disagreements with others, to fail to make your preferences and wishes known, and to fear being assertive, and by doing so you leave yourself open to being manipulated.

You may be pleased when others praise you for being so agreeable. After all, we all get tired of disagreements, hassles, and other unpleasant and upsetting situations. It can be very agreeable to interact with someone who is amiable and congenial. I'm not trying to get you to change being agreeable as this is something you want to maintain. What could be helpful is to reflect on whether or not you have to conceal your real thoughts and feelings much of the time in order to be liked.

It is possible to continue being liked if you voice a different perspective or another opinion. Your likability will not vanish if you want something different from what another person wants. Your pleasant nature will not go up in smoke if you say "no" when you do not want to do something, particularly something someone else want you to do. Furthermore, you can be assertive in other ways. Although there are some people who will not like you when you disagree with their point of view, you will find that there are many who will like you more, and they will respect you.

Reflect on your need to be liked. Everyone *wants* to be liked, but not everyone *needs* to be liked. If you have this need, you may want to work at understanding it better and to become more aware of how it may have been detrimental to your relationships and best interests over the years. Once you become more aware of the extent to which this need may have contributed to unsatisfying and/or destructive behavior, you can begin to make changes. See Chapters 5 and 6 for strategies for change and for guides to greater self-understanding.

Saying Pleasant Things

The belief that people will like you if you always say pleasant things is both valid and invalid. Yes, it is nice to hear pleasant remarks; they can be uplifting and inspirational, and, yes, people will like you. On the other hand, if the situation does not call for pleasantness, your remarks may irritate, offend, insult, denigrate, or be off-putting. You will not necessarily be liked for trying to be pleasant when this situation does not warrant it. In such a case, you are meeting your need to be liked, not assessing the situation and making a more appropriate response. What you may be battling, in part, is the fear that you will be abandoned and left alone. You may want to consider if you are unconsciously reacting to a fear of being alone when you insincerely say something pleasant so that the other person will like you.

Consider having a goal of saying pleasant things only when warranted and that are truthful and sincere. This would mean that you also intend to stop giving insincere remarks and comments and start becoming more authentic in your communications. Becoming more authentic will increase the likelihood of you being liked, even when what you say is not pleasant, because you can be trusted to be truthful, sincere, and genuine.

Taking Care of Others

The belief you can hold is that taking care of others ensures that they will like you and so you put yourself out to take care of others who are capable of taking care of themselves. What is more likely to happen is that you are being intrusive, failing to empower others to take care of themselves, exceeding the limits of your responsibility, and being taken advantage of continually.

Some people will see your helpfulness as a weakness, an opportunity for exploitation, or a signal that you consider the person to be incompetent or inadequate. Some may even think that you have very low self-esteem. At some point, even those nearest and dearest to you will push you away, telling you that you are not needed to take care of them. They can take care of themselves, thank you very much.

You do not want to be indifferent to others' needs and cease nurturing. That would not help you or other people in your life. What could be helpful would be to change the belief that others look to you for their well-being all of the time. Infants and small children would be the exceptions to this. You can become more aware of the limits of your responsibility and engage in self-exploration to better understand what is contributing to your belief.

Loving and Being Loved in Return

"I can feel worthwhile only if I have someone to love me." You may have to dig deep to see if this thought fits you. But if, over time, you have been disappointed again and again by people whom you loved but who did not return your love, then you might consider that you are reaching out to others in the effort to feel worthy.

It is probably not possible to becoming an adult without having thought you loved someone and feeling betrayed and rejected when you were not loved in return or were misled. You may have invested a lot of time and energy in the relationship, only to find that your love was misplaced. The hurt that ensued was deep and difficult to overcome, and even just reading these words may evoke the lingering hurt from that relationship.

Loving someone and being loved in return is indeed a wonderful experience as that can enrich you to feel valued, inspired, uplifted, cared for, and a sense of happiness and joy. Loving and being loved contributes to the meaning and purpose in life and to your well-being, and can even play a role in your physical health. The benefits of loving are numerous. However, when your love is not returned, you can feel diminished and flawed because you did not receive the love you gave to the other person.

If being loved is the only way you can feel worthwhile, then you are missing a number of opportunities to feel worthwhile and may be missing the opportunity to love yourself, flaws and all. There are other ways to feel worthwhile besides being loved by the person of your choice.

Your self-esteem does not have to depend on being loved by a particular person. You can find other ways to love and admire yourself.

Feeling Excited and Alive

"I can feel alive and excited only when I'm with the person I love." Being with the person you love can be exciting and energizing, but if this is the only time when you feel this way, you are investing too much in that relationship, or person, and you may be expecting too much from them and are overlooking other possibilities for generating these good feelings.

Do you feel "dead," empty, or fragmented when you are not with the one you love? If you miss the person, that's okay. But if you have very intense and negative feelings about yourself, that's not okay. These are the feelings that can lead you to act in ways that are not in your best self-interest and may even be destructive. Others can find that it is easier to manipulate you to do what they want you to do when you devalue yourself this way.

Can you remember a time in your life when you felt excited and alive without having to be with a special someone? Was there ever such a time? If there was such a time, you can revive and renew the activities that produced these feelings, for example, dancing, sports, crafts, or volunteer activities to rebuild your energy and self-esteem. If there was never such a time, you will need to create and develop other experiences to produce excitement and energy and explore your early experiences further to find what could have led you to feeling this way.

There are many ways to generate excitement and the sense of being fully alive. These paths are, of course, all personal to the individual, and you will have to find those that best fit you. Now that you have some sense of your emotional susceptibility and have begun to see how it impacts your life and your relationships, we will move to a discussion about how this susceptibility takes place and what you can do about it in the short and long terms.

CHAPTER THREE

Immediate Coping Strategies

The previous chapter presented some material that was intended to help you understand what impact the other person's anxiety may have on you, both short and long term. It is very likely that you are primarily concerned with trying to manage their concerns in the moment, and there are many of these moments, and learning how to better manage these will lessen or eliminate the negative impact on you in the moment and even later. This chapter emphasizes techniques and strategies for the immediate and short term, with some references to the need to build and fortify yourself that will take more self-understanding and practice, and these are presented in subsequent chapters.

The need for immediate coping strategies is for the unexpected and/or unanticipated events and situations that the anxious person in your life present to you. They do not seem to be able to manage what many other people consider to be ordinary or common concerns or problems without resorting to a need to off-load their worries and other anxiety on to someone else, which is you in this case. You are probably not prepared for the onslaught of their negative perceptions and feelings and/or fail to be sufficiently emotionally shielded so that you do not "catch" their feelings. Your emotional susceptibility as discussed in the previous chapter leaves you somewhat psychologically vulnerable to taking their feelings, which can then cause you distress. This can be especially true for close and intimate relationships such as what can happen with the Worrier and Nagger with whom you are close and value the relationship, and in other relationships where your sense of yourself may be touched by the other person's anxiety, such as the relationship with a boss or supervisor who is a Micromanager. However the other person presents their anxiety; the unifying factor is you and why you may be open and vulnerable to that person's anxiety, both short- and long term. This chapter first presents cues to help you identify when the anxious person can be in the throes of anxiety as there may be times when they are unaware of the extent of their anxiety or of their need to off-load some emotional tension. You, as the receiver, may also be unaware of what is happening in the interaction until it is too late to prevent the negative effects on you. So the first section tries to increase your awareness of when the person is likely to be anxious.

The second section addresses strategies to help you manage and cope with the emotional intensity the anxious person displays in the moment that can also help them reduce some of their distress as well as preventing you from catching this distress. The third section addresses how you can manage your responses and prevent emotional contagion. The fourth and final section presents some strategies for what to say and do in these interactions that can be helpful for the anxious person.

Awareness of Their Anxiety

You are likely to be aware when the anxious person in your life is experiencing considerable anxiety even if you don't know the source or reason for their anxiety. They will be exhibiting some of the following behaviors that convey their mental and emotional states:

- Rapid, intense, and/or loud speech.
- Either a rigid body position, or lots of body movement, for example, jogging in place, shifting from one foot to the other, or tapping foot or hand.
- May laugh a lot or the laughter is inappropriate.
- Little attention or time given for social amenities. Will jump right in to talking about their concern.
- Few nonverbal gestures or movements.

It is relatively easy to tell when a child is anxious as they seem to either freeze or to move a lot. It is not as easy to do so with adults as they can try to hide their anxiety from you and others by reducing body movements and controlling their facial expressions. Mostly, however, they are not trying to conceal their anxiety from you, but you may miss some cues and then are surprised when they off-load their anxiety onto you.

What can happen when you are unaware of the extent of their anxiety is that you are caught off guard and are then open to catching their projections and feelings. Your emotional susceptibility and psychological boundary strength determine if you are able to then use your emotional insulation, and either "catch" or ward off the negative effects of their anxiety. Adding to this can be your desire to help the other person, which is admirable and helpful, but the mind-set that you must be of help could be a contributor to your distress encountered in the interactions with the anxious person, and also why you were chosen by that person to be the recipient of their anxiety.

Emotional contagion and susceptibility were discussed in Chapter 2. Your attention to your susceptibility for catching others' projections and feelings and the strength of your psychological boundary strength can be helpful to increase your awareness of the anxious person's level and intensity of their concern whenever you are approached by the person. When your awareness grows, you can then be better able to prevent becoming overwhelmed or enmeshed with that person's anxiety and, in addition, can prevent you from experiencing or carrying their distress after the interaction is completed. You may even be better able to help the person because you can be more objective and not be in the position of trying to care for them and needing to protect yourself at the same time.

Try the Following to Increase Your Awareness

Reflect on a recent interaction with the person you consider a Worrier, Nagger, Micromanager, or Complainer. Try to visualize their approach to you and notice their nonverbal behaviors as they approach you. Notice their facial expressions, walking posture, arms, legs, head, and hand movements. Taken all together, were these conveying tension (rigid, little movement), agitation (lots of movement), or something else? Try to just focus on their nonverbal behaviors, not their words at this point.

As you concentrate on their nonverbal behaviors, try and recall the thoughts, feelings, and ideas or other reactions you had as the person approached you. Can you recall if you were surprised, wary, pleased, or dreading, or had other such feelings? All of these can be helpful for you to learn better ways to cope in the moment. Your awareness of yourself and the other person helps you protect yourself from catching their feelings and projections as well as providing you with alternatives for helping them.

Managing Their Emotional Intensity

First off you can be more helpful if you do not catch their emotions and/or intensity. Once caught, these can be hard to relinquish, so the next strategy is to prevent yourself from catching what they are

experiencing. Three effective strategies for prevention are emotional isolation, eye contact, and body orientation. Emotional isolation was presented
in Chapter 2, and you can launch your wall, force field, gate, or whatever
image you use to isolate yourself from catching their feelings and projections as that does not take much time to use. Eye contact may be harder
in some respects as you may routinely look at them in the eye when you
are talking to or with them. However, when confronted with the anxious
person in your life who seems to be coming your way to off-load their
distress, it is better for you to not maintain eye contact as you are talking.
You don't have to be obvious about looking elsewhere; just look at their
nose, forehead, chin, ear, but not their eyes.

Nonverbal Strategies and Techniques

You may also find it helpful to orient your body away from that person.
Instead of standing or sitting so that your bodies are in sync, turn your body
ever so slightly to the side, and lean slight back. This body position doesn't
have to be obvious, just enough so that you are not fully facing the person.
You are still connected to what the person is saying, but you are not as fully
connected as you would be if you had your body oriented to the person.

These slight nonverbal gestures are designed to protect you while you
are listening to the anxious person and also show that you are aware of
and interested in what they are saying. You don't want to display nonverbal gestures that convey disinterest such as looking around the room or
environment. Managing the anxious person's anxiety as an immediate
response is best done when you can first manage your own response to
their anxiety and not get caught up in their panic, emotional intensity, or
agitation. Your emotional shielding can help with this even when you are
caught off guard and not prepared for their onslaught of emotions.

While they are talking, try turning away from them, or fiddling with
an object, or any other action that may signal disinterest or distraction.
The subtle nonverbal gestures you display probably will not be noticed by
the other person but will protect you, while allowing you at the same time
to interact with them and hear their concerns. This distancing of yourself
from their projections and emotions also allows you to implement more
effective strategies to help them.

Another nonverbal behavior to practice is your voice tone. It would not
be unusual to mimic the other person's voice tone as this can be what
usually happens in many interactions, and you may find that you tend to
reflect the anxious person's voice tone. By tone I mean speed, intensity,
and level of speech—how fast or slow you speak, the emphasis given to

words, and the loudness or softness of your speech. Strive to make your voice tone calm, steady, and softer. You may want to practice the following so that the technique can be easily implemented at any time.

Be conscious of your usual voice tone. Do you talk rapidly or loudly or with emphasis? Are you also breathing rapidly, or holding your breath when you talk? Now, reflect on how you speak when you are relaxed. Is your breath slower and deeper? This is your goal for interactions with your anxious person.

Consciously become aware of your voice tone in the next verbal interaction you have with anyone for practice. As you become aware, also start to try to breathe as deeply and evenly as possible and notice what that does to the pacing in your speech. Also, you can become aware of the emphasis or forcefulness of your speech and, for this purpose, try to soften that emphasis. Steady voice tone that conveys safety—that things are under control, that agitation and panic are not needed, and that you will stay anchored and grounded to help them find their solution. Your reactions can intensify their anxiety or can help reduce it even with your voice tone (even on the phone). The final nonverbal behavior is your facial expression. Just as their facial expression conveys their inner turmoil, so may yours give away what you are thinking and feeling. Your facial expressions can be better controlled if you do not maintain eye contact as described earlier, and make sure that your body is turned slightly away so as to prevent emotional contagion. Your goal for your facial expression is to have it reflect that you are listening, open to what they have to say, and reserving judgment at this point. Depending on the relationship, such as that with a micromanaging parent, spouse, or boss, you may not want to have a neutral facial expression. You may find it best, regardless of the relationship, to not look alarmed, surprised, irritated, or apprehensive. Although you may find it difficult, you may also do not want to want to look too welcoming, especially if you have other current responsibilities, tasks, or places you need to be in. You are trying to convey the anxious person that you will take some time for them but that you are not inviting them to linger and linger and linger.

Distractions

Don't forget that the anxious person in your life can have an urgent and important issue, concern, problem, or crisis that needs immediate attention. Even though many or most of the concerns or problems that they bring to you may be urgent only to them and their anxiety is a usual response to even trivial matters, don't assume that everything is, and make your judgement about the importance and seriousness of the matter after hearing what that is. When the matter your anxious person brings to you is not urgent, not vitally important, trivial, or not relevant to their existence or current well-being, you can try to use distraction as a means to calm them down, by thinking instead of feeling; to encourage them to think of their own solutions; or to even get them on a more productive topic. All of these reasons can also assist them to reduce their anxiety.

Distractors should be used to pull them away from the emotional intensity around their current concern, which can then provide you and them with sufficient time and space to collect your thoughts. You can quickly plan your strategy, launch your emotional shielding, and manage your breathing. Examples for distractors can fall into the categories of manners, breaking news, the environment, flattery, and the like to give you suggestions for how to think of some that may help you.

Manners mean that they would probably want to respond in a way that was not rude or otherwise unacceptable. They would need to be cordial and to respond to what you are saying first before voicing their immediate concerns. Start with a greeting like "Good morning," but don't add "How are you?" Instead, say something like, "It's shaping up to be a (busy, eventful, lazy, relaxing) day for me!" Good manners would require that they respond first to what you said before jumping into relating their concern. Use the surrounding environment as a distractor such as the weather, for example, "Good morning (afternoon, evening)! Isn't this a great day weather wise?" Or, "Isn't this downpour miserable?" (the environment can be the room, office, or restaurant, or wherever you are to provide a comment that will act as a distractor).

Breaking news as a distractor would be something like, "Good morning, have you heard about _____?" Try to make that news about something pleasant and meaningful to you or them if possible, or just of passable interest. One example would be, "Did you see where the local baseball team is having a winning season?" It's not necessary that either of you care deeply about that subject, just enough to use it as a distraction.

Flattery is a comment about the anxious person, for example, what they are wearing such as "That color shirt looks good on you," how their appearance is such as "You're looking well this morning," or "I don't know how you stay so well and on top of things." Say something from their world would get their attention for enough time, it will let you get ready to manage your and their emotional intensity. The weather is usually safe to comment about, if at work, the traffic, asking if the trip was uneventful—any room can provide material for a distraction and you can capitalize on numerous environmental items. Flattery, when used in a reasonable way, can provide distraction. It can be about something in the present or in the past, about appearance or actions, or something you appreciate about the other person. It is the rare person who does not respond in a positive way to a flattering comment. If the anxious person does not respond or seems to dismiss your comment, that can be a clue that whatever is causing the agitation is very serious for that person.

On the other hand, there are some actions you want to avoid as distractions:

One-upmanship where you describe that your woes are greater than theirs are

Sarcastic comments about their concerns, especially those that seem to minimize or dismiss their concerns

Long stories that provide lots of detail but are meaningless

Telling the anxious person about someone else's problems in an effort to get them perceive their problems as lesser or of no importance

These and other similar actions can distract the anxious person but do not contribute to maintaining a cordial relationship. Following are two additional strategies that may be helpful.

Movement—Take a Walk

It could be helpful to both of you if you could stroll while talking. The act of walking could be calming as well as providing opportunities for distractors. You can suggest that the two of you take a short stroll for more privacy or that you might be able to listen better, or that there will be less noise or something that will allow you to better attend to the person.

Moving can give you time to think about managing their intensity and to use your emotional shielding, both of which can be helpful when attending to their anxiety is unexpected. The content of their concern, problem, or issue is less important than is their emotion and its intensity as this is what fuels their anxiety and your possible distress. It is not that the content is unimportant as it may well be important; its more that you are chosen as a resource to take away some of their emotional intensity as realistically you are not able to solve it, fix it, or change it in most instances. Just the simple act of walking can help provide some respite and time so that you can more effectively provide the reassurance they seek or use your plan for coping with their anxiety.

Redirect to Cognitive Matters

There are times when your anxious person can be lost, enmeshed, or overwhelmed by their fears, worries, or problems and concerns that increase their anxiety and make it difficult for them to function. Of course it is at their most intense when they seek you out and tell you what's producing their anxiety.

Another constructive technique is to *redirect their focus* to cognitive (thinking) matters away from their current emotionality. This doesn't mean that you ignore their emotions, as these carry an important message about them and play an important role in the interaction. It does mean that the cognitive focus has the potential to reduce some of the intensity, which, then, allows them to better manage their own anxiety.

Redirecting can take the form of asking a question that calls for thinking, for example, asking about the possible options they considered for solving the problem, taking action, or identifying the major barriers and constraints. Another form could be presenting an option or alternative phrasing it as "Have you thought about _____?" Another redirect can be reinforcement of a previous thought or action such as "I remember when something similar was happening to you and you _____. What seems to be different now that what you did before would not work?" Basically, a redirect should be related to the present concern and not a change of topic. Other lead-ins that can be used to redirect their attention could be as follows:

How do you plan to _____?

What are some significant barriers and constraints that you've thought of?

What do you need more information about?

What do you think led up to this?

Getting them to think instead of becoming overwhelmed with their feelings can help calm some of the anxiety as well as guide them to create their own solutions.

Immediacy

Presented were some immediate techniques and responses that you can implement when the anxious person in your life approaches you unexpectedly and you have taken by surprise with their concern and emotional intensity. To summarize, immediate techniques and strategies use the following:

Employ your emotional insulation

Use nonverbal positions and gestures to prevent catching their emotions and its intensity

Identify and insert distractions

Move to another location or take a walk

Focus their attention on something cognitive

Plan as discussed in Chapter 4

The final suggestion is that you keep some part of your attention on your breathing to help keep it calm, steady, and deep. This can be helpful because your calmness in the face their emotional intensity will allow them to catch some of your calmness and lower their distress. Following this section are some goals for immediate responses, some actions to avoid, suggestions for getting to the core of the matter, and other ways to manage the interaction.

Managing Immediate Interactions

There are four primary tasks for constructively managing immediate interactions: prevent emotional contagion, determine goals for this particular interaction, actions to avoid, and finding the core concern. There are more strategies and techniques, but usually immediate interactions don't give you time to think through those and to select the best at that moment. However, if you can remember to focus on these four tasks, you will find that you will be effective in managing immediate interactions.

Prevent Emotional Contagion

An effective strategy to help manage interactions is to first use your emotional insulation. This bears repeating because you can forget to do this when unexpectedly confronted with another person's sending or projecting their intense feelings. While it can be best to have it already in place, you have probably experienced several incidents where the interaction and its intensity was unexpected, but it can still be effective when you are belatedly using it.

One way to develop your emotional insulation is to visualize something between you and the speaker such as a wall, gate, curtain, force field, or anything that will screen and keep their emotions out while allowing you to continue to hear what they are saying.

When in interactions with your anxious person and you feel their emotional intensity, you can immediately think of the barrier you use as emotional insulation: a curtain, a wall, a gate, or whatever will work for you. A quick visualization like this that usually takes seconds can help prevent you from catching their feelings that are usually somewhat intense in the moment. You will be more effective and helpful if you are able to do this.

Goals for Short-Term Interactions

It is helpful to have some goals and objectives for interactions in the immediate present. You may want to think of these in advance so that you are not trying to manage your emotional reactions, their emotional intensity and trying to understand their concerns at the same time. What are some possible goals and objectives for the immediate interaction?

1. Manage and reduce your and their emotional intensity
2. Prevent catching their distress
3. Understand their issue, problem, or concern
4. Soothe their distress
5. Manage their panic

Prioritize and Work on one goal at a time.

As you read these examples, you may think that all or most of these are the goals for any particular interaction. What I suggest is that having too many goals or objectives is not effective or helpful as you cannot work on all of them at the same time and trying to do so can add frustration. Just think about a recent interaction that was frustrating or distressing for you and reflect on whether some of the frustration could have resulted from you trying to do too many things at the same time. While all of these can be done in an interaction, they are more effective when done sequentially instead of jumping from goal to goal. What follows are suggested steps and techniques for creating priority goals and objectives for immediate interactions.

1. Use your emotional shield.
2. Manage and reduce your emotional intensity, discussed earlier in the chapter. Make a conscious effort to breathe deeply and to employ your emotional insulation if not already in place.
3. Understand their issue, concern, or problem as they perceive it. While you may see a pattern, deeper issue, or concern, or even possible solutions, it is also possible that you are interpreting something they don't mean or intend. It is also helpful for you to understand their perspective and to verbally reflect this back to them. This simple act can be somewhat calming for them. You can show this understanding of their perspective by repeating the concern or rephrasing it in your words, or summarizing what they said.

4. As they are talking, you can use the speaking time to judge if the concern or problem is one of the following:

   a. Urgent and important—Crisis or almost a crisis. Immediate action needed.

   b. Important but not urgent—Immediate action is not necessary and there is time to consider and choose the best options or alternatives.

   c. Urgent—Usually this is their urgency but may not need immediate action.

5. Sometimes their urgency is communicated as panic. If they are in a state of panic, a calm soothing voice when you respond is helpful. However, it is also important that you do not minimize their concerns as a means to reduce the panic or some of the other actions to avoid, which is discussed later in this chapter. My strategy for managing panic (mine or others) is to reflect on:

   a. Am I dying—usually not, so no action needs to be taken. If there is danger or concern, and the answer is yes, then immediate action needs to be taken.

   b. Is someone else dying—If there is danger or concern, take immediate action. If the answer is "No," then move to item c.

   c. Do I need to take immediate action—If the answer is yes, then act appropriately. If the answer is no, then you have time to think and plan how best to handle the situation.

Actually, the process of thinking about each of a, b, and c generally calms me so that I can be more effective.

These are realistic goals for immediate interactions.

Actions to Avoid

Whatever your goal is, the following are not recommended. You may find that these are impacted, but it is best to not have these as immediate goals.

- Soothe their distress—Your calm behavior and matter-of-fact attitude can be soothing, as would breathing. They may become soothed in the process of talking to you, but that will be a desired outcome, not the goal itself.

- Provide solutions to their issue, problem, or concern—This is also desirable but somewhat unrealistic as you may not fully understand what is causing their anxiety, which is manifesting itself as unrealistic and unnecessary worry, resulting in micromanaging, nagging, or complaining. You cannot help solve whatever the current concern may be as it goes deeper, and your solution would not address is not their real or underlying issue, problem, or concern.

There are also some other actions to avoid such as

1.   Saying "Calm down" or something similar
2.   Platitudes
3.   Trying to use logic or get them to use logic while they are emotionally intense

"Calm down"—This is a phrase that is more likely to increase their emotional intensity or arouse their anger. Yes, you are correct in thinking that if they calm down they would be able to feel less distress and think through their dilemma. Try to respect that they are unable to calm themselves down at this time or they would have done so. In some instances, saying "Calm down" is like pouring rocket fuel on a small fire. That only helps intensify it.

Platitudes are not helpful, as these do not demonstrate any understanding whatsoever about them or their concern. Platitudes are a message to your anxious person that you don't want to hear their concern, don't want to have to deal with their intensity, do not care that they are upset or even about them, and so on. Platitudes convey indifference about the other person. If you are interested in preserving the relationship, you will refrain from using platitudes.

Logic will not be helpful either because they will not be able to follow it as you present it. The logic is yours, not theirs, and what seems logical to you is not necessarily logical to someone else, especially someone who is anxious about their concern, and trying to get the anxious person to be logical may only frustrate them and increase their emotional intensity.

Words will matter in these immediate interactions. Your anxious person already feels inadequate and can be very sensitive to even the slightest hint of criticism or blame. It can be important that you carefully choose your words to be neutral, or affirming of the person, or to show that you have confidence in their ability to deal effectively with the issue, problem, or concern, or in some situations to find the help that they need. Just listening sometimes is what is helpful for the anxious person.

Your solutions are unlikely to work for someone else as you are very different from others. It is probably best that you do not give advice or provide your solution for their concern. You may be able to see alternatives and/or options, and it is best to present them with the caveat that what you are seeing as possibilities are your perceptions and thoughts, and that there may be others that you don't see or think about.

Presented were some techniques and strategies to help manage immediate interactions with your anxious person. Next are some additional techniques and strategies that can be used to get to the core of their immediate problem or concern, set reasonable time boundaries, and examine more effective and efficient questions.

Finding the Core Concern

Managing the emotional intensity of the anxious person in your life, in addition to trying to manage your emotional susceptibility, is very challenging but can be done if you will be able to focus your attention and theirs on the core concern, issue, or problem. The emotional overlay can be so intense and pervasive that either or both of you may not be able to discuss the core concern. What follows are some suggestions that can be helpful to use in the immediate interaction to get to the core of the matter. These are not presented as steps as it may not be possible to use them sequentially. The basic objectives are to identify the primary issue, and distill it in few words.

Identification of the primary issue, concern, or problem can be challenging for many reasons: their emotional intensity, your emotional intensity and susceptibility, how the immediate concern is presented, the relationship of the two of you, your understanding of the anxious person and knowledge of their history and personal characteristics, the environment where the interactions occurs, and other such variables. Try to distill the volume of words they use to describe the concern or problem into as few words as possible. That can sound daunting but can be really helpful. For example, many issues, concerns, or problems for these anxious people arise from their fears about their adequacy or perceived adequacy, or of falling short, or some vague dire consequences. Whatever their concern is about specifically, it will generally revolve around some unspoken fear about their ability to cope or manage. You'll see this even when the spoken concern is about another person in that the underlying concern is about the anxious person.

To help them to identify the core concern in a few words, try to get them to state the issue in six words. There are times when more than six words will be needed, but many core concerns in a problem can be stated in six. Try the following to understand what is meant.

Think of a current concern you have and write it in six words. Let's say that you overspent last month and are now worried about making ends meet. Stating or thinking the concern in six words might look something like this:

Overspending
Fewer funds
Bills
Budget crunch

The last two words define the problem succinctly. Let's try another one. Your Micromanager boss is once more checking on your progress using your valuable time needed to work on the task. The concerns of the boss can be stated as follows:

Incomplete task
Encourage completion
Check progress

So, no matter what the boss asks, the core concern is the status of progress. In both examples, you can use the last two words to cut through the verbiage and emotional intensity and restate the basic concern in a couple words to show understanding. That can also reduce the time needed for a particular interaction.

More Effective and Efficient Questions

Do not ask "why" questions as these are not helpful. Why questions carry an implication that the person is inept, or to blame for the problem in some way. The anxious person is emotionally intense, and why questions do not lead to solutions or resolution and can be irritating to the other person. Examples of what not to ask are like the following:

Why don't you try to think this through?
Why did you do what you did?
Why don't you just _____?
Why is this worrying (bothering etc.) you?
Why do you keep doing that?
Why is this important to (do, you, think about)?

You may think that you are helping with the why questions, and, in some instances that could be the outcome. However, much of the time, "why" isn't helpful.

Instead of why, try just reflecting back their current concern and let them talk. Unless you want to spend a lot of time on their concern, asking for explanations, probing for information, or providing suggestions with the why questions will significantly prolong the interaction and can probably increase their distress.

Manage Your Reactions by Boosting Your Mood

There may be times when the interaction with the anxious person in your life leaves you in a depressed mood and this may linger for some time. Following are some reasons for thinking about and developing mood boosters as a way to moderate your reactions.

- Develop a set of mood boosters. Tips for developing some are found in the appendix. No one strategy will fit everyone or will work every time, or even be appropriate for every event. Indeed, what worked for you at one time may not work for you at this time. This is one reason why you need to have a set of mood boosters, be open to adding new ones, and be flexible in choosing which to use at any particular time. Place and time can also be factors for using effective mood boosters.

- Do not suggest mood boosters for the anxious person in your life. You may be tempted to try and boost the mood for your anxious person in the effort to make them feel better. It is best to remember that each person is unique and that your mood boosters may or will not fit anyone else. If you do have an urge to be helpful, try asking the person what usually works for them, and gently suggest whatever work be tried now, or if that is not possible at this time, ask what other actions the person thinks might be helpful.

- What do you have on hand or around you that could be used to boost your mood? You may not be aware of the resources you have or that are around you that will boost your mood. Many people may not realize or recognize resources they have available all around them and so fail to use these and remain mired in the negative mood. What can be helpful is for you to identify your unique sets of mood boosters, create and try new ones.

- Understand that you can boost your mood and that your mood boosters come from within you and are not entirely dependent on what another person says or does. Whatever your mood may be at any particular time, it is related to your inner essential self and how you perceive and feel about that inner essential self. Hence, what works to boost your mood lies within you.

- Become aware of when you may be catching another person's mood as it is possible to catch others' moods. Emotional contagion was discussed in Chapter 2 and is also relevant here. To understand how this can work just think about how you feel at the times when you have to interact with someone who is sad, mad, or happy. You may find that you too have become more in tune with that person's feelings and have started to have some or all of that feeling too. That process is called emotional contagion. This can also happen when you interact with your anxious person and catch their mood.

The major assumptions are that you can manage and control your moods and that there are mood boosters that can be low or at no cost to you. What is presented here are guides to help you develop your personal lists of mood boosters that can be used at any time when you have a negative mood, such as what can happen after interactions with your anxious person. You have numerous mood boosters all around you that are quick and that cost little or nothing. Yes, there are some grand mood boosters, but those usually take planning, time, and money and may not be readily available at the needed moment in your life. You do not have to wait as you can boost your mood at any time with just a little thought and effort, and with little or no cost to you. In addition, there are other added benefits for using mood boosters.

Benefits

The benefits to you for preventing negative moods from emerging, or for intervening when these do emerge, can be significant. The effects for both positive and negative moods can be experienced in your body, in your relationships, in your mental processes, in thoughts about your self, and even on your ability to function. There can be times when you try to let go of the negative mood, or to get away from it, but are not successful or worse, you engage in acts that are not in your best interests such as overeating, drinking alcohol to excess, buying things that you don't need or may not want, or other such activities, some of which can be self-destructive. The mood boosters you think of or create should be designed to give you more constructive alternatives for getting out of a negative mood or preventing one from emerging and are intended to be encouraging and supportive of a positive mood. Benefits include the following.

- It is in your best interests to boost your negative mood, given the substantiated mind-body connection.
- Relationships can be improved.
- Thought processes can become clearer, problems are seen as capable of being solved and solutions created, and ideas emerge.
- You can feel better about yourself.
- Increased ability to tolerate and work through little barriers, problems, and the like.
- Increased enjoyment, pleasure, and appreciation.
- You are more apt to be able to visualize success.

The Mind-Body Connection

Negative moods can produce body stress, and stress, especially prolonged stress, can have negative effects on your body and your physical and mental health. An occasional negative mood is not likely to have much physical effect, but having more frequent ones could produce health-related problems such as sleep difficulties, over- or undereating, extensive use of alcohol and/or other mind-altering substances, high blood pressure, and other such problems. Having few such negative moods and being able to reduce or eliminate their duration can lessen the bodily stress that can result from negative moods.

Reflection: Reflect on the state of your health and health habits and assess the extent of your satisfaction with these when your mood becomes negative. Are you more or less satisfied with how your body responds to negative moods?

Impact on Others

Other people in your life can also experience an impact resulting from your moods, either for a negative mood or for a positive one. It is reasonable to expect that others, just as you do, have their moods affected by your moods, not only those who are close to you but sometimes even people with whom you have limited contact. Boosting your negative moods could lead to improved relationships.

Reflection: Recall the last time you had a negative mood and how that may have impacted other people who are closest to you. Is this what you intended?

Clarifies Your Thoughts

When you feel down, distressed, or irritable, or have some other negative mood, do you find that it is more difficult to concentrate on the task, think through a problem, generate ideas, stay focused, and complete other such mental functions? Some people do find that their thought processes are affected and that they tend to be more focused on personal concerns or to have chaotic thoughts switching from one thing to another. This can help to produce a downward depressive spiral. Boosting your negative mood can produce clearer and sharper mental functioning and interrupt or prevent the downward spiral.

Reflection: How are your cognitive processes affected when you have a negative mood? Would you characterize your mental state as sluggish, easily distracted, hard to maintain focus or something similar? Contrast that with how you are able to think, plan, concentrate, and the like when your mood is positive.

Better Tolerate Barriers and Constraints

The world continues to present you with challenges, problems, and barriers (these can also be termed "little annoyances") when your mood tends to be negative. It can feel as if the world is conspiring to make you feel worse. Examples can include things similar to the following:

- You cannot reach the person you need to give you the information to solve a problem.
- Unexpected roadwork or an accident makes you late for work or for an appointment.
- Your alarm clock did not go off or was not properly set.
- You or a family member go to the emergency room.
- What you had planned to wear is not clean.
- Rules, guidelines, and the like change or are modified without prior notice.

In addition, your energy and other inner resources can feel depleted so that you are not as able as you usually are to work through these. It is also possible for some people that they can become more irritable or more withdrawn when in a negative mood. Acting to boost your mood allows you to better assess these challenges, problems, and barriers; to seek out strategies to address them in a constructive and productive way; and to be creative in addressing these.

Reflection: When are you most able to work through problems, barriers, and challenges; when your mood is positive or when it is negative?

Increase Positive Feelings about Yourself

This is a major topic that is explored throughout the book, and only an introduction is presented here. Everyone has feelings about themselves regarding their competencies, abilities, self-worth, self-efficacy, lovability, and other such characteristics.

Negative moods can affect these feelings about yourself, and, instead of focusing on your positive competencies, abilities, and so on, you start to focus on and become distressed over what you consider to be your faults, mistakes, shortcomings, and other such negative things. Once begun, it becomes difficult to stop as one negative thought or feeling about oneself seems to lead to another and another. Some people continue to follow these thoughts and feelings to the point where they begin to entertain self-doubts, leading to feeling that they are fatally flawed and shameful. Boosting your mood at any point during this process can help prevent intense negative feelings about yourself.

Reflection: Try to recall your general mood when you last berated yourself, blamed and criticized yourself, or felt inadequate. Was your mood negative before you had these self-thoughts? Did your mood seem to make these thoughts about yourself worse?

Enjoy Your Life

A major positive benefit for mood boosters can be your increased enjoyment, pleasure, and appreciation for what you are and have. You benefit in many ways when you have these positive feelings, physically, cognitively, and relationally. Getting out of a negative mood allows you to see and appreciate the positives in your life, and doing this allows you to function better.

Reflection: Let a memory of a day or time when you were happy, felt pleasure, or appreciated something or someone emerge, and re-experience how wonderful that felt. Allow yourself to remain with that feeling for a few moments or even longer.

Visualize Success

Boosting your mood permits you to visualize success mostly in all aspects of your life. You become better able to see possibilities, alternatives, and options, and to imagine solutions. Your thought processes are clearer, you have the energy to act in your best interests, plus you can have more zest and enthusiasm to work toward success whatever that may be for you.

Reflection: Make a list of three successes you've achieved and three that you want to achieve.

Summary

There are steps and techniques that you can take to minimize the negative impact of the anxious person's emotional intensity when you are taken by surprise by their need to express their concern(s) and do so with extensive emotional intensity. The unexpectedness of their presentation can make it a challenge to maintain your equilibrium, to prevent catching their emotions and their intensity, and to think of ways that you could be helpful. Presented were some strategies and actions that you can find helpful and descriptions for some actions to avoid as these are not helpful and have a potential for making things worse for you and for them.

CHAPTER FOUR

Advanced Preparation: Let Others Have Their Feelings

Sam was sitting in the family room when his wife came home from the PTA meeting very upset. He asked what was wrong, and she spent the next 20 minutes telling him how the president of the PTA had ignored her suggestions, had been contemptuous of her, and did not understand anything. As she talked, she became even more upset and angry, and Sam found that he too was becoming angry. He started pacing the floor, clenching his teeth, and balling his fists. As he became angrier, his wife calmed down. Sam "caught," identified with, and acted on his wife's anger.

People who have an emotional or psychological investment in others' well-being can often be very sensitive and responsive to others to the point where they are open to catching others' feelings without recognizing that this is what is happening. On the other hand, people who are powerful senders of their emotions are described as being relatively insensitive and unresponsive to others, especially other people who are responding to them. What seems to happen is that emotionally susceptible people are open to the emotions of the other person, but the senders are either closed or indifferent to the emotions of others.

To put this concept in person terms, there may be instances where you may attend to and care about the other person's feelings, wants, desires, and/or needs while the other person is interested only in getting what they want, regardless of the cost to you. In such a case, your caring and concern is used against you.

Senders have some common characteristics that you may recognize. They are frequently:

- Nonverbally expressive
- Exploitive
- Powerful projectors of emotions
- Able to recognize and exploit vulnerability
- Acting from strong power, control, and manipulative needs
- Able to lie, mislead, or distort to get what is wanted
- Relatively unempathic

The Dynamics of Nonverbal Expressiveness

Nonverbal behavior is thought to be more expressive of true feelings than verbal behavior in most human interactions, and it is said to carry 90 percent or more of true messages. Most nonverbal behavior takes place on the unconscious level, and both the person exhibiting the behavior and the observer send and receive the message on an unconscious level. This unconscious level makes it more difficult for you to be consciously aware of what is being acted out at the time it occurs.

Thus, the dynamics of what can happen are these: You may have a psychological investment in the other person; that person wants something from you; you are open to receive their nonconscious, nonverbal message on your unconscious level; and you then respond unconsciously to the message. The unconscious nature of the nonverbal communication and response may startle or surprise you and leave you bewildered about what happened.

Let's try to examine what takes place on the nonverbal level. Because you already have a psychological investment in the other person, you are more likely to trust them and to feel that the two of you have some rapport. The types of relationships where psychological investment is expected to be mutual are these: parent-child, married partners, lovers, and relations between family members. These would be the strongest, closest, and most intimate relationships. You may have other relationships, such as close friends, that are also characterized by your psychological investment in the person. The degree of trust and caring, of course, will depend on the particular relationship and the person.

When you trust someone and feel that there is mutual rapport, even when there is evidence to the contrary, this can mean that your nonverbal behavior communicates receptiveness. This receptiveness is indicated nonverbally in the following ways:

- Making eye contact
- Leaning forward
- Orienting your body toward the other person
- Mirroring the other person's posture
- Holding your arms by your sides
- Removing barriers between you, for example, a sofa pillow, touching or allowing yourself to be touched
- Concentrating visibly on what the person does or says

In this way, once you are attending to the other person nonverbally, you are then open to their projections and projective identifications.

Senders use nonverbal gestures, like those described in Table 4.1, which can reflect their intent.

In order to counter the sender's intent, you can increase your ability to recognize their nonverbal communication, identify your nonverbal receptive behaviors, and institute changes for your nonverbal postures and gestures. These can then become a part of your emotional shielding to make your messages more powerful and accurate. Specific suggestions and strategies are presented throughout this chapter.

The latter part of this chapter presents some specific strategies for recognizing the sender's nonverbal communication, identifying your nonverbal receptive behaviors, and changes for your nonverbal postures and

Table 4.1 Gestures and Messages

Gestures	Intent
Making eye contact	Establish connections, rapport
Looming over you	Intimidation
Touching you	Power and control over you
Orienting their body toward you: "cornering"	Manipulation, seduction
Mirroring (reflecting your gestures and body positions)	Seduction, establishing rapport
Moving closer	Make you feel "in sync," merged, or enmeshed

gestures that can become a part of your emotional shielding. Your messages can become more powerful and accurate.

Exploitation: Senders and Receivers

Some senders have considerable underdeveloped narcissism (see Chapter 3), which can lead them to exploit others. Of course, they do not see it that way. They are unaware and uncaring about their exploitive behaviors and consider it their right to manipulate others into doing whatever they want. It will be helpful for you to understand that these senders do not have much complete understanding of their own psychological boundaries, that is, where they are separate and different from others. These people are still operating under this mistaken, infantile perception that other people are only extensions of themselves, and thus under their control. Children experience this a lot when their parents think of them as extensions of themselves.

These self-absorbed people are taking care of their "self" at all times. Even when they use words that seem to indicate an awareness of others in the world, you need to be aware that this is only a surface ploy, and it is done to accomplish something for their own good, not yours. All of their acts are in the service of the self.

This may be a difficult concept to accept. However, the extent to which you can reduce or eliminate your emotional susceptibility largely depends on your recognition that you are operating under faulty assumptions. You need to develop more realistic assumptions; for example, senders are always looking out for themselves first and foremost.

One difficulty you may experience when trying to recognize and accept the trust that a particular person is exploiting you is that the exploitive person usually has some very engaging characteristics; for example, they are charming, persuasive, and attentive. Such people can make you feeling special, valued, lovely, and worthwhile, and these are wonderful feelings. For example, when your mother says something that makes you feel she loves you, you may feel uplifted, even though you know she is saying it to manipulate you. We all like these feelings, and we are drawn to people who make us feel that way. However, if part of what happens in a relationship results in you feeling or being exploited, then you are paying too high a price for the wonderful feelings.

There are also senders who exploit other people by inducing feelings of guilt and/or shame in them. (Parents are very adept at this.) When you are involved with these senders, you wind up doing things you do not wish to do, and you feel exploited because you were told you "should" or "ought" to do those things. The induced guilt and shame results in you carrying out the sender's wishes.

Exploitation consists of both external and internal assaults. Someone wants something from you, and they do or say something that triggers an internal responsiveness within you, and you then act to provide the person with what is wanted. You must understand what your triggers are if your emotional shielding is to become effective. But, first, you need to recognize that although the sender is exploitive, that they do not know that they are exploitive, and that this person generally feels that they have a right to use you and others in service to their "self."

Powerful Projectors

Some people are powerful projectors of emotions, and it can be very difficult to block the emotions they project, even when you are not in a relationship where you have psychological investment in that person. For example, actors earn their living by projecting emotions to audience. You have no connection with them, they are playing their roles, and you can still end up feeling the projected emotion. Children are also powerful projectors. The younger they are, the more powerful their projections can seem. If you are not shielded, you can easily feel the emotions that infants project.

The projectors in your life, however, who are cause for concern, are neither actors nor children. The senders who are causing you distress are using their feelings to manipulate you into doing what they want you to do. You are not reacting out to your independent desire; you are feeling the brunt of that sender's feelings and reacting to those feelings. Remember, for both of you, this manipulation takes place on the unconscious level. You are not consciously aware of the sender's projections, and that person is not aware that they are projecting.

The more primitive emotions of fear and anger also tend to be the most powerful ones, and you are probably reacting to these most of the time. To illustrate, suppose you are with someone who is a powerful projector, and they want you to do something but are not sure you will cooperate. This person unconsciously feels that (1) they are entitled to get what I wanted; (2) have a right to expect and/or manipulate you to give what is wanted; and (3) are *fearful* of not getting the need met.

What can happen is that the sender's fear is projected onto you, and the sender then reacts to you as if you were fearful, for example, moving closer, using a soothing voice, or caressing or patting you to reassure you that you need not be frightened. You react to the fear by trying to "make it all better" by accepting the unwanted soothing and denying your real feelings, thus addressing the projected fear. If the sender can keep you from expressing fear, then they do not feel that fear, but you continue to carry that fear.

Your reaction and feelings are much more intense if you identify with any or all of the projected fear. You incorporate that fear, make it part of yourself, and then become manipulated by it. This is another example of projective identification. Your psychological and physical boundaries have been violated, and you are not consciously aware of the intrusion.

Exploiting Your Vulnerability

Other people can sense your vulnerability. Unknowingly you may send out signals that indicate you are available for manipulation and exploitation. I know that seems like a harsh statement, but it is important for you to increase your awareness of how you may contribute to some of your own distress. Your insecurity; lack of confidence; spongy, brittle, or soft psychological boundaries; your need for connections and reassurance; and your desire to be loved and valued put you in apposition where others can sense that you are open to manipulation and exploitations. Add this to your conscious desires to be a caring, thoughtful, considerate, and sensitive person. Such desires are commendable but not helpful in your present circumstances.

What are some of the signals you transmit that help the senders to sense your vulnerability? They might be nonverbal behaviors such as the following:

- Fingers in your mouth, or hands over your mouth
- Shifting eye contact
- Slumping posture
- Entering a room tentatively and looking around
- Holding your body closed in on itself
- Speaking in a very soft voice
- Smiling at everything, everyone, or a lot

Some verbal indicators you might use that indicate your vulnerability are the following:

- Using qualifiers that might make what you say tentative and unsure
- Being indecisive

- Raising your voice at the end of sentences, which makes it seem as if you're asking questions instead of making statements
- Seeking others' approval
- Not asking for what you want, but waiting for it to be provided for you
- Agreeing to keep the peace
- Talking about failed relationships

It may be pleasurable to be liked for others seeing you as shy and sweet, but the same characteristics that indicate shyness and sweetness are often seen as vulnerabilities.

Power, Control, and Manipulation Needs

Three different types of power and control need are discussed here: they are coercion, reward or reinforcement, and referent. Coercion relies on threats, intimidation, and other use of force to exert power. Reward or reinforcement uses the promise of real or psychological goodies to exert power. Negative reinforcement, that is, the threat of withdrawing something of value, also falls into this category. Referent power is the power you bestow on the other person. That is, you decide that the person has status, charisma, or a powerful personality, and your perceptions give that person the power that can then be used to manipulate you. For example, in high school, the status awarded to the captain of the football team and to the Homecoming Queen gives them referent power. The process used to get what you want from others, which involves the use of one or more power and control strategies, is called manipulation.

Coercion is easy to understand as a power behavior. The other person is forced in some way to do what is wanted. Force can be any of the following: persuasive arguments, appeals to one's desire to be cooperative or liked, group and peer pressure, and the use of physical force and verbal threats. If you respond to any of these, you will want to make your objective, eliminating your openness to being coerced.

Reward or reinforcement power uses tangible and/or fantasized goods and services to gain what is wanted and to manipulate others. Positive reinforcement is putting something in, like a present or promise of future goodies. Negative reinforcement is taking away something desirable that is believed to be present like affection or financial support. Your responses to such power plays illustrate your needs and vulnerability. If you are fearful of losing someone's attention or affection, you will respond by giving that person what they want. The same is true if you are desirous or needy of attention or affection.

Review your current and past relationships of concern, and note which ones are distinguished by power and control as their salient characteristics, especially those where you were coerced. Power and control are especially characteristics of many family relationships.

You will want to examine your particular needs that made you susceptible to the power and control needs of others. You will also want to examine those relationships where you bestowed power upon the other person.

Lies, Distortions, and Misleading Statements

Senders make considerable use of lies, distortions, and misleading statements to manipulate you and others. These people do not have any sense that their dishonesty is morally wrong; they are just "doing what everyone else does." Many of their lies are of the variety called "white lies" or "sweet lies," where the sender's intent is to make you feel good. When you feel good, you are more likely to appreciate them and do what they want you to do. Many people consider lies like these harmless. They do not realize the negative impact such lies may have.

You, and some senders, may engage in flattery, insincere comments, compliments, and other verbal acts that are less than honest. This is not to propose that you should always be brutally honest. "Brutal," by definition, can be very hurtful. This is just an attempt to show you that you, too, act in this way, and there is seldom any malicious intent. You did not set out to hurt the other person. A sender, however, may feel the same way consciously but, unconsciously, may want to manipulate you for personal gain.

Making yourself immune to flattery is certainly one way to stop being manipulated. Needing to hear flattery, compliments, or "sweet lies," for example, "I could never love anyone but you. You're the only one for me," contributes to your emotional susceptibility. Do you respond to statements like the following by feeling valued, pleasured, or appreciated?

- No one understands me like you do.
- You're the most beautiful (handsome) person in the world.
- I don't think I can live without you.
- You're a better daughter (son) than your siblings.
- Just looking at you makes me feel good.
- You've got something no one else has, and I like it.
- You give me something no one else can give.
- You understand me in a way that no one else does.

There are relationships where any of these statements is a true expression of feeling. What you must learn is how to distinguish when such statements are "sweet lies" and when they are honest feelings. This is not always easy to do. Your need to be flattered, complimented, and told "sweet lies" should be a part of your self-examination.

You cannot stop others from lying, distorting, and making misleading comments. What you can do is to better understand the psychic payoff when you hear such comments. This deeper understanding of your own responses can lead to being able to distinguish between white lies and an honest expression of feelings and lessen your need for flattery and compliments. You can reduce your tendency to be manipulated significantly by increasing your understanding of your need to be flattered.

Lack of Empathy

It can be hard to accept that anyone is insensitive to your feelings. However, senders tend to lack empathy, and until you can accept them as they are, that is, insensitive to your feelings, you will not make much headway in developing emotional shielding, and you will stay open to "catching" their feelings.

You may find it difficult to see senders as they really are because you make the faulty assumption that they are, in many respects, like you. After all, there is support for the idea that we feel understood by people with whom we share common characteristics. Since you probably consider yourself as a caring, considerate person who is sensitive to others' feelings, you may operate on the unconscious assumption that the people in your world, or those to whom you are attracted, are similar to you in this respect. This assumption will be one of the most difficult fantasies you have to overcome.

You probably have ample evidence that some people in whom you have a psychological investment (people like your parents, siblings, and other family members) are insensitive to your feelings and/or the impact their behavior has on you. Yet you continue to expect them to change, any minute now. But they do not change. They continue to be insensitive. These are the people who:

- Push you to do what they want
- Refuse to accept "no" for an answer
- Don't recognize when you are upset
- Change the subject if you try to talk about your feelings

- Redirect all conversations to focus on themselves
- Use all the right words, but the feelings behind the words are absent
- Have an essential coldness at their core
- Are ruthless in pursuit of what they want to get
- Feel entitled to have what they want, regardless of the cost to others

You may be defending yourself from recognizing their insensitivity by rationalizing, repressing, or denying both the person's behavior and its impact on you. Nothing you can do or say will cause this person to change. Nothing. If the person changes, it will occur because they perceive that changes are needed and desired. The only constructive acts you can take are to work on yourself: build resilient, strong boundaries; develop emotional shielding; and engage in a more realistic appraisal of the people in your world and your acceptance of them.

Shielding against Emotional Assaults and Projections

Building a shield against external forces will take some effort and require you to make some changes in your habits. There are very effective nonverbal and verbal strategies to help repel emotional assaults from others, protect you from their projections, and give you more time to work on your shielding from internal assaults. As you read through the next section, select the strategies you feel are in accord with your personality. When you first begin using any of these, you will probably become uncomfortable, but stay with your plan. At some point, your discomfort will cease. Your goal of building strong, resilient boundaries begins here.

ACTIVITY 4.1 YOUR FIRST SHIELD

Materials: Felt markers, crayons, or colored pencils; two large sheets of paper 18 × 24 inches.

Procedure:

1. Sit in a quiet private place with a desk or table for drawing. Close your eyes and imagine you have a shield in front of you. Notice every detail about the shield on both sides, the side facing you and the side facing out. Observe the height, length, width, density, the material from which it is made, color, decoration, and so on. This shield can protect you from others' emotions and projections and is being developed for you.

2. Imagine how far the shield is from you. Is it six inches or closer? Further than six inches? Is it touching your body? Where is it?

3. When you have a good picture of your shield in your mind, open your eyes and draw it on the first sheet of paper, noting as many details as possible.

4. On the second sheet of paper, draw a picture of yourself with your shield in place. Try to place the shield the same distance from your drawn figure as you imagine the distance when your eyes were closed.

Look at both pictures. You can recall these anytime you need to remind yourself to put your shield in place. Be patient. There will be times you will forget to use the shielding, or remember it only after someone has ignored or breached your boundaries. The trick is to learn to raise your shield before the emotion assault and/or violation takes place. That will take time, practice, and conscious thought.

This activity is entitled "Your First Shield" because there is more work to be done to fortify this shield and to build strong, resilient boundaries for yourself. For a first step and for the short term, this shield will suffice.

Nonverbal Strategies

There are nonverbal strategies that can be more easily instituted than anything else, and when used judiciously, they will allow you to make more independent and objective decisions. You can lessen the effect others' emotions and projections have on you when your nonverbal behavior gives you the space to move away and the time to think instead of feel, to analyze, and to evaluate what is happening. Your actions then can be guided by careful consideration of your options rather than by impulsive reactions to emotions.

Changing your nonverbal behavior can be very powerful since the nonverbal component of message is the most accurate. One reason you have been the target of others' emotions and projections is that you nonverbally convey receptivity and vulnerability. Here are two exercises.

Incorporating Nonverbal Strategies into Your Shield

You have begun to build your external shielding. You now have some ideas about where your personal and intimate comfort zones are located, an image of your personal shield, and some sense of how your body and gestures may communicate receptivity. You have received some suggestions, for example, moving your social and intimate zones further back, and many more suggestions are forthcoming.

However, before suggesting additional strategies, let's take a look at the circumstances where you most often become enmeshed or overwhelmed by others' emotions. There are numerous situations where this might happen, and it can be helpful for you to understand better where and when you seem to be most vulnerable.

- Do you become enmeshed or overwhelmed quickly and without warning?
- Do you realize only gradually that you are enmeshed or overwhelmed?
- Is it only after evidence of betrayal, abuse, or other insensitive acts that you accept that you are enmeshed or overwhelmed?
- Are you ever warned by others that you are letting someone get too close or that you are being manipulated, but you don't see the relationship that way?
- Are you convinced that you can help the other person?
- Do you wake up one day and realize that you've become enmeshed and/or overwhelmed again?
- Are you readily available as a "shoulder to cry on"?
- Do you want to see the good in everyone so much that you ignore or overlook behaviors and attitudes to the contrary?

The first two questions may provide some guidance for short-term strategies you can use. If the "catching" of emotions and projections happens quickly, you will want to examine the settings where this occurs. For example, does it generally happen in social situations where you are trying to have a good time, and you are not on guard? Social situations can be especially vulnerable places and times, as can family gatherings. You are generally sociable and outgoing during these times and willing to overlook or deny any concerns you may have about a relationship, and this leaves you open and receptive to "catching" emotions and projections. Understand where and when you are vulnerable can help you become more aware of staying shielded.

If the "catching" of emotions and projections happens over time, and you become aware of it only gradually, the strategies you would use are different than when the "catching" is quick. You would need a blend of external and internal shielding to deal with a gradual awareness, whereas quick "catching" can be addressed with external shielding only. However, even when you awareness is gradual, you can use external shielding to give yourself the space and time you need to reflect on what is happening, your responses, and possible pitfalls.

Nonverbal Shielding against Quick Emotional Catching

The following section presents some nonverbal strategies you can use to shield against the quick "catching" of others' emotions and projections. Review these first to determine whether you do the opposite behaviors, such as making eye contact. Then, read the list as a cluster of gestures and behaviors to be instituted almost in their entirety, at first. As you gain stronger and build more resilient boundaries, you can relax using some of these clusters for you will have a better understanding of when to allow yourself to become connected, and to whom.

- Do not attend to the other person such as orienting your body to them.
- Do not sustain eye contact; look at the person's nose or forehead.
- Move away ever so slightly.
- Restrict smiling or mirroring the other person's facial expression.
- Entwine your legs.
- Look around the room.
- Visualize somewhere else, for example, a place of peace.
- Don't preen, that is, don't stroke yourself, nor fiddle with your hair or jewelry.

Do not given the other person your full attention or act interested in what they say to the exclusion of anyone or anything else in the area. Look around, turn your head away, and orient your body away from the person as if you are leaving or inviting others to join you. If standing, move back a few inches; if sitting do the same or put something, like a purse, between you. If you have to look at the person, restrict your smiling or mirroring of their emotions and do not maintain eye contact.

Suppose you have an uncle who always tells you all of his woes in exhausting detail, and you end up "catching" his feelings. You like your uncle, but you want to stop catching his emotions. Think about your physical stance, your posture, and so on, when you tend to "catch" his feelings. You probably stand close to him, your body turned (oriented) toward him, you sustain eye contact, and your facial expression is sympathetic or similar to his. To stop catching his emotions, you can alter your physical stance as described earlier. These body and facial shifts do not have to be major changes even minor adjustments will help.

Let's try on a harder situation. You suddenly realize that your aunt is well on her way to seducing you to do something you do not want to do. What she specifically wants you to do is not as important as the fact that you do not want to do it. Your thoughts and feelings are confused and complex because you want to maintain the relationship, please her, and not arouse her anger or your guilt, but you don't want to do whatever it is that she wants you to do. The discussion about internal forces (see Chapter 6) will try to address your thoughts, feelings, faulty assumptions, and so on. As noted before, these are more difficult to address. The focus here is only on extracting you from the situation so that you do not wind up doing something you did not want to do.

If you follow the behavior described earlier and physically move back, break off eye contact, stop mirroring her facial expression, and repeat to yourself, "I don't have to do anything I don't want to do," you can disassociate yourself. Unfortunately, your aunt will most likely be the type of person who continues to push to get her way, regardless of what your nonverbal behavior may be communicating. You may need to give up your fantasy of being subtle and become more direct, that is, more even further away. Visualizing your external shield will also be helpful.

Verbal Strategies

Your nonverbal behavior will be more effective when combined with one or more of the following verbal behaviors:

- Do not explain, use excuses, or use other signals that you are being defensive.
- Do not respond.
- Do not argue.
- Use a clipped, strong voice.
- Use titles and be formal when addressing the other person.
- Say "No" and leave, hang up if on the phone, and so on.
- Tell the person that you don't appreciate their attempts to manipulate you.
- Propose that you and the other person take some time to get to know each other.
- Say, "Get away from me!" if a less direct approach fails. This is unlikely to be misunderstood.

When you *explain* or provide an excuse, other people can perceive this as defensiveness and that you are susceptible to manipulation, seduction, or exploitation. *Not responding* is classified under verbal strategies because various ways of nonresponding are used that relate only to verbal exchanges. That is, the person who is trying to seduce, manipulate, and/or intimidate you is using words, and your tendency may be to respond to words with more words.

You may be tempted to *argue* with the person or have the erroneous idea that you have an obligation to respond to whatever is said to you. You do not. You have no obligation to *reply, explain, argue, or defend* your position, or to even answer their questions. Too often, when you respond, you only provide another opportunity to the sender to send you emotions or projections that you can then "catch."

If you are in the habit of using a *soft, quiet voice,* try to save that voice for special people and for special occasions. Speak in a *clear, decisive voice* that is moderately soft. You can always soften your one to sound "sweet," "sexy," or soothing. It's much harder to raise your voice after starting to speak softly. A strong voice conveys confidence and self-assurance and sends the message that you intend to take care of yourself.

Do not remain in the other person's presence after you say "no." Say it clearly and firmly, and *then leave,* or, if on the telephone, *hang up.* Staying available gives the person another opportunity to try to change your mind, or it may convey the message that you are ambivalent and that some possibility exists for you to change your mind. Whether you are right, wrong, or indifferent about saying "no," when you say it, stick with it.

There are more aggressive verbal strategies to use if you need them. These illustrate going on the offensive. For example, you can *tell the other person* that you recognize what is happening, and you do not like it. You may receive the response that your perception is wrong, but the person will back away. In addition, you have indicated a strong sense of your boundary. That is always a good thing to do.

At first, these strategies may seem rude to you, and you may have some reluctance to use them. However, if you are not being respected by the other person, you are the only one who can save yourself. You needn't be rude, but there are some people who get the message only when faced with an aggressive statement.

Blend Verbal and Nonverbal Strategies

The third set of strategies is a blend of verbal and nonverbal approaches. This set includes behaviors and attitudes such as the following:

- Do not discuss your personal concerns except with trusted confidants.
- Hear only meaningless noise when someone is trying to manipulate or seduce you.
- Do not ask for favors except from a few trusted people and rarely do so with them.

- Visualize the person in a comical or undignified situation or position.
- Be indifferent to what they are saying.

When you *discuss your personal concerns*, you tend to focus on your feelings about these concerns, thus leaving you vulnerable and open to "catching" others' feelings. You can become mired in either positive or negative feelings and forget to maintain your boundaries. You are distracted and focused on yourself at this point which means that others can use your distraction as an opportunity to project their feelings onto you, and your defenses are not in place to prevent you from "catching" them.

You may yearn for comfort and reassurance, and because the other person is saying what you want to hear, you make the faulty assumption that they care about you. What the other person perceives is that this is a golden opportunity to seduce or manipulate you. Be very selective about the people with whom you share your personal concerns, and try never to share personal concerns in social situations.

You do not have to *listen to or hear them.* I once saw a cartoon that showed a man talking to a cat. The man was telling the cat that her behavior (the cat's) was unacceptable. The balloon above the cat's head indicated that what the cat heard was gibberish—meaningless sounds. Yes, the cat was attentive, but kitty didn't hear or understand one word. Trying to imitate a cat and not hearing or understanding what the sender says to you can be a very effective strategy.

Do not ask others to do favors for you except when to do so is unavoidable. Make sure you really need whatever is requested and do without whenever possible. When others do us favors, there is an implied or a direct expectation that we are under an obligation to return the favor.

There are people in this world who prey on others by doing favors for them and thus making them feel obligated. Such favors never seem to be adequately repaid. And such people never let you forget that they did a favor for you. If you did favors for others, let them be gifts with no expectation of payback.

When you start to feel that you are "catching" emotions or projections from others, you can pull yourself back from being caught by visualizing the other person in a *comical situation or position.* Visualize the person in situations such as these: dressed in a clown's costume or wearing a dunce's hat; stuck in an undignified position like receiving a pie in the face; and so forth. It's hard to catch an emotion or projection when you are secretly laughing inside.

Indifference is a powerful tool against "catching" emotions and projections. Indifference is like a dense gray fog that nothing can penetrate. You simply do not care. It is not your concern or problem and you have no intention of trying to "fix it"; neither are you going to anything to try to make the other person feel better. Learn how to act indifferently even when you do not feel indifferent. When your internal shield is better fortified, you will be able to be appropriately indifferent in reality. Care when you want to, but do not care to the point where you become enmeshed or overwhelmed by others' emotions.

CHAPTER FIVE

Increase Your Effectiveness: Become More Helpful

The discussion to this point has focused on how you can prevent becoming distressed in interactions with your anxious person. We now move on to suggestions for how you can, at the same time, become more helpful and effective. After all, you do want to show your caring and concern even if you cannot fix the concern for the person, give solutions, or make their problem or issue or concern disappear. Presented here are techniques for managing your emotions and eight response categories that can be effective for both of you. Chapters 8 and 9 present suggestions for interacting with the specific category of anxious person: Worrier, Micromanager, Complainer, and Nagger. What is presented here are general responses that can be used judiciously with all of them, or selectively as they fit you, the other person, and the situation. Also presented and discussed are some actions and attitudes to avoid as these are counterproductive for meaningful and enduring relationships.

An essential component for increasing your effectiveness and at the same time being more helpful is your ability to manage your emotions. While you may be outwardly seen as controlling your emotions, and that is important, it can be even more important for you to also understand these and be able to lessen their internal impact.

Managing Your Emotions

Managing your emotions means that you are aware of your feelings in the moment and do not think or feel that they are appropriate to express at this time, or that you are more effective when you are guided by your thoughts rather than reacting on the basis of your feelings, or that your feelings seem out of sync with the situation. Your reasons for trying to manage your emotions are valid for you and are irrelevant as it is more important that you learn how to manage your feelings than it is to identify why you have or need to manage them. Managing also means that you are not repressing or denying these feelings and, while there may be some suppressing for the moment, you are doing so because it is not in your best interest or that of another person to express or act on them.

There are some self-reflective steps you can take in advance to prepare yourself to better manage your emotions so that when intense or distressing emotions emerge in a situation or interaction, you can think about what to do and not just react. This will enable you to be more in control of yourself and of the interaction or situation. The first step in getting ready to manage your emotions involves accepting responsibility, understanding the role of self-statements, and the associations you have with previous events and persons.

Getting Ready—Accepting Responsibility

Preparing yourself in advance for interactions and situations where your intense and negative feelings may be triggered starts with accepting responsibility for what you are thinking and the feelings you are having. All too often some people will blame the other person for their personal feelings with thoughts or statements similar to "You make me so angry." The hidden messages in such statements are the following:

You should not do or say anything that triggers my anger.
You are wrong (bad) to trigger my anger and you should be ashamed (or punished).
You must (should, or ought to) take care of me and not trigger my anger.

Blaming the other person for what you are feeling is not helpful and shows that you are not accepting responsibility for your feelings. Yes, what they said or did or failed to do were triggers for you, but the real responsibility for what you are feeling lies with you. Your task is to understand why these feelings were triggered, not to bestow blame and criticism on the other person. It is very helpful to accept that you have feelings for a reason, but not that someone caused or is causing you to feel the way that you do.

Getting Ready—Self-Statements

When your negative feelings are triggered, a primary source is your self-statements. Self-statements are the thoughts and feelings and beliefs you have about your core and essential self. Many feelings such as guilt, shame, anger, and fear can be triggered by your self-statements. Guilt is usually what is experienced when we think that we have failed to act in accordance with our values and standards. While these may have familial and cultural roots, we can continue to use these as the expectations for how we act. Shame emerges when we consider ourselves as fatally and deeply flawed to the point where we cannot get better or be healed. We work hard to keep our shameful self hidden. Anger is the reaction to perceived danger, and we need to get ready to fight or for flight. Fear is the reaction to the possibility of immediate destruction, and that we are helpless to prevent that. These are uncomfortable and intense emotions that most people experience. There are also graduations for these feelings, such as embarrassment as a milder form of shame, and those are less threatening to have as our feelings than are the more intense forms. These feelings can be a source for negative self-statements.

Sometimes when your negative feelings are triggered by your self-statements, these are the statements you feel to be true under the present circumstances. You don't have these thoughts and feelings about your self all of the time, but there can be times, circumstances, interactions, people, and the like where you may unconsciously think and feel these about your self, which then leads to you experiencing the negative feelings.

Following are some self-statements that can produce negative feelings. As you read the statements, try to recall a recent or past situation or interaction where you had intense and negative feelings and ask yourself if you also had one or more of these self-statements at that time.

- *I'm inadequate, and I can't do anything to please.*
- *I'm incompetent, and I can't do anything right.*
- *I'm shameful and not fit to be with others.*
- *I will be abandoned and left alone.*
- *I will be destroyed (emotionally, relationally, figuratively, or even literally)*
- *I cannot take care of myself, and I need others to take care of me.*
- *I am powerless to control what happens to me.*
- *I am hopeless and cannot get better.*
- *I am helpless and unable to do what needs to be done.*

You may have found as you read these statements that you did have some of these thoughts about yourself. For example, you may have felt helpless in an interaction with your anxious person or hopeless or inadequate at meeting their needs, demands, and so on. Understanding the possible causes and associations for the self-statements will be addressed later in this chapter. Right now it is helpful to identify if and when you may have these self-statements that can contribute to your negative and intense feelings.

Getting Ready—Identify and Assess the Threat

Negative self-statements can erode your self-confidence and self-efficacy. You're less competent and effective when you feel angry, ashamed, guilty, or fearful. It can be helpful for you to identify and assess what is happening in that moment that produces these feelings and the accompanying self-statements. Of course, I am not referring to situations that are physically dangerous. What is meant here are those situations and interactions where you don't feel there is physical danger, such as in interactions with your anxious person. However, lurking in any situation or interaction can be a possibility of psychological danger to yourself. This is what is meant in this section—either consciously or unconsciously you may sense a threat to your psychological well-being that may be valid or not. Your self-statements are not based on the validity of what you sense; they can be irrational and invalid or real and valid. However, you do have the negative self-statement and one way to manage your feeling in the moment is to identify what in the situation or interaction may be contributing to your negative self-statement, for example, what is taking place in the here and now that is triggering your self-statement, "I'm inadequate."

The next step would be to assess the validity of the self-statement on a scale of 1 (no validity) to 10 (considerable validity). The validity index can give you some idea of the reasonableness of your self-statement and the accompanying feeling. Let's suppose that your self-statement is about your adequacy and your validity rating at this time is 2, and the accompanying feeling is guilt. The questions to ask yourself would be how reasonable is it for you to think you're inadequate (the 2 rating) under these circumstances and then to feel guilty. On the other hand, suppose your rating was 7 or 8, and you assessed the validity of the rating. It would be more reasonable to have some guilt feelings if you felt this inadequate. It may be best to put the self-statement and the resulting feeling aside for the moment and analyze them later. What you may want to focus on and gather information about is what is it in the present situation or event that seems to have triggered the self-statement, and to block the negative feelings you are having. You can explore your feelings later.

When you get more experienced at thinking about what is happening in the moment, you can also consider the possibility that you are catching projected feelings from the other person in the situation or interaction. If you are possibly catching their projected feelings, then part of what you are feeling is a result of their negative self-statements that are adding to those you have. It may even be that your feelings were not as intense when you started interacting with the person as they are not. All of this may all seem very complex and may be confusing. Another point to remember about all of this is that neither you nor the other person are aware of what is taking place as this can all be on an unconscious level: your self-statements, your feelings, and their projections that are adding to your feelings. Most likely, you are consciously attending to the content in the interaction and thereby catching their feelings which is on the unconscious level. Once you identify and assess the threat to your self, you can use your emotional insulation to prevent further catching and make a mental note to explore your self-statement and feeling(s) later when you can do so without intrusions or disruptions.

Getting Ready—Change Your Self-Statements

The previous section presented the impact and roles for negative self-statements you may have that get triggered by interactions and situations with your anxious person. The self-examination process referred to in that section will be presented later. We now move on to another strategy you can use in advanced preparation. That strategy is to change your self-statements, but you first have to identify which ones you have. The goal is to develop more logical and realistic self-statements that you can substitute for your negative ones. Following are some logical, rational, and positive self-statements that you can substitute and, after examination, adopt in place of your negative ones.

- I do have adequacies and strengths and I need to remind myself of that.
- I can do many things correctly and adequately.
- I try to live up to my standards, and I will continue to grow and develop regardless of mistakes and setbacks.
- I have meaningful and satisfying relationships, so I will not be alone. I will work to make these better.
- I may be hurt by some actions and comments, but I will survive.

- I can take care of myself.
- I have power over some things, but mainly I have power over myself.
- I am realistic in my hopefulness, and I will not lose my hope.
- I am capable in many ways, not all, but some.

You may need to practice your positive self-statements to reinforce your belief in them.

Getting Ready—Examine your Self-Statements

Many of your self-statements arise from one or more of the following sources: parental messages and relationship, family-of-origin experiences, and other past relationships. Parental messages are those thoughts and feelings you internalized about your self that came from your parent(s) figures. They directly and indirectly communicated to you how they perceived you as valued, worthwhile, and loveable as well as how they perceived your other personal characteristics such as your intelligence, looks or appearance, personality, and the like. The negative self-statements you have could have their roots in those old parental messages that you still carry and act on.

Reflection: Find a place where you will not be disturbed and sit in silence and breathe deeply for a little while. Allow yourself to recall a significant negative self-statement, and if that statement is a reflection of messages your parents/parental figures either directly or indirectly communicated to and about you many times. Then, reflect on the validity of that message about you today. For example, let's use the self-statement about your adequacy. Think about the ways today that you are adequate or demonstrate adequacy. Now, rate the validity of that old parental message about your adequacy today. You will likely find that the old parental message about your adequacy no longer fits, or has been modified in other ways. See if you can let go of some or all of the old message and strengthen the new one that you are adequate by reminding yourself of the many ways that you are now adequate.

Some family-of-origin experiences may also relate to your negative self-statements, and these can be explored as were the old parental messages. You may have had experiences with siblings or other relatives that also communicated their perceptions of you, and you may have internalized some of these and accepted as being true about yourself that are still influencing you today.

Reflection: Recall on your family-of-origin experiences that immediately come to mind when you start thinking about them. The experiences you recall do not have to be in chronological order; just let them emerge as you think about the messages about yourself embedded in these experiences. If you like or think it would be helpful, you can write them on a sheet of paper. As you compile your list, ask yourself about the validity of those past and current family-of-origin messages. You may wish to try and discard or dismiss those that are not valid today. Another exploration that could be helpful is to reflect how or if those old messages are reflected in your self-statements, and how they could be related to your triggered feelings. Is it possible that you are reacting to the new relationships and interactions or situations based on those old family-of-origin experiences and messages? If so, then you may want to reinforce your positive self-statements.

The last associations that may hold some understanding for you may be found in some of your other past relationships those with other people who were influential in helping to shape your growth and development. Their interactions with you also provided you with messages about how you were perceived, valued, and appreciated. Review the previous two reflections for parents and family and substitute other influential people you recall. It could be that some or all of the self-statements and/or your feelings emerge from past associations with some of your past relationships.

Concluding

Managing your emotions is critical for a more effective communication with everyone in your world, and understanding why you feel and react as you do is the basis for managing these emotions. Once you associate your current feelings and reactions with old messages and relationships, you can be better able to recognize when your responses in the present may be more about your associations with the past than they are objectively and rationally about the present. Just this understanding can reduce or eliminate some of the intensity and negativity you may be experiencing.

Seven Responses to Reduce Their Anxiety

In addition to managing your emotions, you need some effective responses and strategies to use with your anxious person, and these are more effective if you know what you want to do in advance for interactions. Even better is when you can practice them in advance. Following are seven responses that can be effective:

- Moderate their emotional intensity in the interaction
- Distract their attention

- Blur the nonessentials
- Restate their essential concern
- Provide a blank slate
- Focus on content
- Calm the frenzy

All of these responses are provided with the understanding that the relationship is important to you, that you do have some caring and concern for the other person's welfare, and that you do want to be helpful if you can. Helpful for this discussion only means that you want to reduce some of their anxiety, not to fix their problem, issue, or concern. Each response can be used intentionally to help the anxious person to better focus on the primary or core concern at the moment and to guide them and you to use thinking instead of getting mired in feelings. This also allows time and space to take calming breaths *without* saying anything that suggests the need for them to calm down, all of which can work to reduce the emotional intensity for both of you. In addition, use of any of these strategies gives you the opportunity to employ your emotional insulation.

Moderate Their Emotional Intensity

A good response is a direct attempt to moderate the anxious person's emotional intensity. What usually happens is that you notice and/or catch the intensity and want to lessen its impact on you and so you try to get them to become less intense. Saying things like "**you're really emotional,** or calm down, or take a deep breath, or what's got you so stirred up" and the like are either not helpful or very much less effective than the suggestions presented here. Remember that we are not talking about crises as those that call for very different responses. The anxious person here is anxious about everyday ordinary things, actions, people, and the like. Whatever that produces anxiety for them is usually not as serious as would be a crisis.

So how can you try to moderate their emotional intensity? First and most helpful is to attend to your physical reactions and make a conscious effort to breathe deeply and talk calmly. This will not only help you stay centered and grounded, but the anxious person can begin to mirror your breathing and respond to your calmness. You are conveying a sense of caring, concern, and confidence. Next, make your first statements that reflect good manners, civility, and courtesy. No matter how overwrought or intense someone is, they will stop and respond to a greeting such as

"Good Morning." I've noticed that even when someone greets me, such as saying "Hi" or "Hello" and I respond with "Good morning (afternoon, evening), they then always again respond with my greeting. They say "Good morning" in return even though they have already greeted me. Most people have learned good manners at some point in their lives and will tend to respond to your good manners. This strategy too gives them the opportunity to reduce their emotional intensity.

Another strategy you can use depends on your anxious person and the relationships. That is, you can take a couple of minutes to engage in chit-chat, either about you or about them. Nothing long or involved, just make a pleasant conversation. An example could be something like, "My garden is doing well this year. I'm pleased by its productivity." Don't get caught up in the chit-chat and start to supply details, it is just a statement that is about something other than the anxious person's concern at the moment.

Chit-chat could also be a compliment about the anxious person, such as the flattering color of a piece of clothing, the hair style (this works for men too), or jewelry; a comment they made at a meeting, or something that they do well. The final suggestion is to ask a question about nothing of consequence that can also interrupt the emotional intensity but does not detract from their concern. Examples could be as follows:

How do you think the project (event, planning, task) is going?

Watched any good programs on TV lately?

Did you see the performance?

How do you manage to do so much?

Do you know of a good store where I can find _____?

Now, you certainly don't want to engage in chit-chat when the other person seems to be having a crisis, but for everyday and/or ordinary concerns, chit-chat gives you some small amount of time to breathe. Manners, breathing, and chit-chat can be helpful at times.

Distract Their Attention

In addition to the techniques for moderating emotional intensity, distracting the anxious person's intensity can be helpful. The anxious person tends to be almost entirely focused on their concerns to the point where that is the only thing they are aware of, and this seems to increase their anxiety. Distracting their attention can help moderate some emotional intensity for both of you and allows them time to think, reflect, and review mentally the concern that is triggering their anxiety.

Distractions are all around you. Look in the immediate vicinity and notice what can be used as a distraction, such as one of the following.

- Attending to traffic
- Noticing barriers to walking or standing, such as "Watch out for the high curb"
- Physically uncomfortable searing
- Dodging other pedestrians, skateboarders, and the like
- Unusual signs, clothing, hair styles
- Sayings on T-shirts
- Pleasant or unpleasant odors
- Sounds and/or silence
- Pets, children, and the like

Other kinds of distractions can be used as the intent is to provide a pause. It is helpful to try and think of what could be one or more distractions for your anxious person in advance knowing that at some point you may need them. Preparing now will permit you to have something readily available. You will not have to try and rapidly think of something when you are in the moment with the anxious person.

Blur the Nonessentials

Many, if not all, anxious people tend to present you with many nonessentials when trying to get you understand why they are anxious, or that the situation is dire and catastrophic, or that they just don't know what to do and you have to provide the answer or solution. It is very easy to get sidetracked and caught up in nonessential details, which take a lot of time to communicate, more time to understand, and then even more time for you or them to determine the core or essential issue. There is also the possibility that what you consider to be essential is not what the anxious person thinks is essential. However, it can be helpful to try and focus on what you think are the essentials in the immediate issue, problem, or concern.

One guiding principle is that it is the anxious person's feelings about the matter that is an essential component, and not necessarily the content or actions about the matter. Thus, if you can help the person identify their feelings about their matter, you can begin to help them blur the details and save some time. Some possible nonessentials to be on the lookout for are the following:

Details about what was said and by whom

Explanations about why this matter is important or why an action was taken, especially actions taken by someone else

A history of what led to the current situation

The anxious person's in-depth thoughts about the matter

It may be necessary to interrupt the person, and you may struggle with interrupting as it is considered rude to interrupt. But there are gentle ways to interrupt the detailing and story. Start with an apology for interrupting, such as "I'm sorry for interrupting." Then use something like one of the following:

I'm getting lost (or confused) with the details.

This is more information that I can take in at this time.

I think it is more important for me to know how you are feeling about this matter.

What do you consider to be the most important for you to think about (act on) at this moment?

It seems to me that your major concern is _____.

Some details, explanations, history, and the like might be necessary at times, but, for the most part, these are not very relevant to the anxious person's current concern.

Restate Their Essential Concern

Whatever the anxious person's essential concern may be, it may be helpful and clarifying for you to restate it. That way, the person knows they were heard and understood gives them an opportunity to correct any errors in what was said or what was heard, to clarify any misunderstandings, and to keep the focus on the essential concern. Because of their emotions, many times it is not clear to you or to them what the core issue is, and when you restate what you perceive to be the core issue can be just what the person and you need to help them gain some perspective.

It might be safe to say that the core issue is almost always about their adequacy in one form or the other. The Worrier is concerned about preventing or coping with the matter. The Micromanager is concerned about their adequacy to get you and others to complete the task or job so that they will be perceived as adequate by others. The Nagger is much like the Micromanager in some respects as they think that their adequacy may be called into question when they cannot get you to do what they think is necessary. For example, the home keeper may worry that friends will not consider them to be adequate if they can't get you to always pick up your clothes. The Complainer can be concerned about their adequacy in ensuring that everything is perfect. Of course, this is not'how they perceive their concerns, but at the root of their anxiety is their apprehension or fear that they will not be perceived as adequate or that, indeed, they are not adequate. This fear about self-adequacy makes it easier for you to discern the core issue regardless of the lack or multiplicity of details they provide.

You will not want to say any of that to your anxious person as doing so is likely to produce defensiveness or denial. What you can say is something like one of the following:

"Do you see the core issue as something over which you have control?"
"It seems to me that you are doing the best that anyone could, given the circumstances."
"It is frustrating when others don't have the same (goal, perspective, understanding) that you do."
"You are trying to ensure that everything gets done (on time, properly, etc.)."

Since the core issue is likely to be about them in one form or the other, restating and affirming your confidence in them to manage and cope with the situation can be helpful. Such responses are not minimizing or devaluing their distress; these are the sort of responses that acknowledge the distress without judging if it is right or wrong, or good or bad.

Provide a Blank Slate

There may be times or an anxious person's intrusion where you don't feel that you are up to dealing with their concerns and especially their feelings. You may be trying to cope with a personal immediate concern, when you are suffering with a medical condition, or have urgent and important things to take care of at home or at work, or there may be other reasons why you cannot give the anxious person in your life the care and attention they are seeking. You may not want to cut them off, or can feel that you must listen to them and be polite, or other such reasons where you cannot just walk away. Providing a blank slate could be an acceptable option.

The blank slate is your face and responses where you seem to be indifferent. You hear, you respond, you may even ask questions, but you are not responding from your usual position of caring and concern for the person or for their situation. They can tell you whatever they want to, but your responses are neutral. You may appear to agree, but your responses could also be perceived as you are not having an opinion. Examples for indifferent or neutral responses are "Really," "Uh Huh," "You don't say," "How about that," "I see," and "You do have a point." These are responses that do not carry a judgment about the correctness or appropriateness or of any kind of evaluation, encouragement, or support. The neutral response may not be what the anxious person is seeking, but it is also hard for them to challenge. In addition, because of your current state, the blank slate and response may be the best that you can do at this time.

Focus on Content

Because of the relationship you have with the anxious person in your life, you may be more inclined to focus on their emotional intensity when the interaction is initiated, but there are times and reasons to focus on the content, not the feelings. For example, there are some people who find that it intensifies their feelings when they talk about them. So, when you say something that recognizes their feeling, they think that you want them to talk about the feeling, but, as they talk about it, the feeling becomes more distressful and intense for them. You do not want to increase the distress or intensify their feelings.

Reflection: Visualize an interaction with the anxious person in your life and recall if they become more emotionally intense as they talk about a feeling, especially a negative feeling. Then, try to recall interactions with the person and if they usually become more distressed and intense as they talk about their concern and feelings. Recall if they will say something to suggest that talking about the concern is getting them more upset. If so, then you will want to do as suggested earlier and focus on content.

Another reason for focusing on content even though the feelings carry the main and most important message is that doing so gives both of you the opportunity and direction to think instead of getting mired in the emotional intensity. You can return to the feelings later. Just like what was presented in the section "Restate the Essential Concern," you can reflect and/or restate the core cognitive concern. Let's try to give some examples for the types of anxious people.

A response that focuses on the cognitive is in quotes.

The Nagger who wants you to remember to do something—"Remembering to do something seems to be easy for you."

The Complainer about a paper delivery—"You like to be able to count on something being consistent."

The Micromanager about a task—"Being updated on my progress lets you know I'm on the right track."

The Worrier about something going awry—"You want to anticipate possible problems."

As you read these examples, you may become aware that the concern the anxious person has does have a basis in reality, is expressing something of value, or could be helpful under some circumstances. Reminders and remembering is important, having consistency and reliability is comforting, and not wasting time by making mistakes or going in the wrong direction or preventing problems are all positives. By focusing on this content, you affirm your anxious person's core or essential concern, which is helpful to the relationship. While you may wish that they didn't feel compelled to nag, complain, micromanage, or worry so much, and to share all of this with you as often as they do, you still recognize the nugget in their concerns.

Calm the Frenzy

Some anxious people can get in a highly agitated state that seems to feed on itself and take over their ability to think, to talk logically and rationally, or to even be aware of another person. They become caught up in whatever is fueling their anxiety to the point where they cannot articulate what is going on with them. They can talk fast, have jittery body movements, wave their arms and hands regardless of who or what is in their vicinity, jump or move from foot to foot, and give other such signals of agitation. There is a frenzy of pointless activity. If you want to be helpful you can try to calm the frenzy. But, first, you have to make sure that you are not catching their anxiety and that your emotional shielding is firmly in place.

Here is a sequence you can use to think about what to do when the anxious person is in a frenzy. It goes like this. Mentally consider the following.

1. Is the anxious in danger of dying or of immediate medical or other help? The answer is usually, "No." If the answer is yes, then the action is to take care of them. This becomes your number 1 priority for thinking and acting.

2. Determine if the frenzy is about someone else is dying or in danger. First, ask them if someone is dying or in danger of dying, and if the answer is yes, then take immediate action, such as seeking help, calling 911, and the like. If the answer is no, and most often the answer is no, then move to the next step.

3. Ask yourself and the anxious person, "Does this have to be handled, or any action taken right now?" If the answer is yes, then the two of you can begin to explore and decide what action is best to be taken at this time. If the answer is no, then you don't need to take action.

By the time you've worked through this sequence for yourself and with the anxious agitated person, both of you are usually calmer, are more in control of your emotions, and can think more clearly and logically. All of the agitation is not eliminated, but the anxious person may now be in a place where they can better explain what is producing the agitation. Of course, taking calming breaths throughout the sequence is helpful for you and can serve as a model for the anxious agitated person.

CHAPTER SIX

Their Anxiety: Some Causes

Let's take a look at some of the possible causes for their anxiety that leads to worrying, micromanaging, nagging, and/or complaining. As you read about this, you may want to also reflect on how your experiences are similar and how they may be different. By noting these commonalities, you will be better able to understand why they react as they do, gain insight into your responses to their and your anxiety, and thereby create more effective ways to react and respond. The primary topics covered are the dynamics of their inner world, some life experiences and the faulty assumptions that can be planted throughout life, possible self-absorbed behaviors and attitudes, and what they do not or cannot see about themselves.

Dynamics of Their Inner World

Their inner world referred to here consists of their thoughts, feelings, and the resulting ideas about their meanings. Some of the anxious person's inner world is known to them; they are conscious and aware of these aspects and influences on their outer actions. There are other parts of their inner world that are sensed but not fully known or do not appear in their awareness. And there is a part that is unknown to them and may not yet be accessible but could be accessed, and then there is a part that, in all probability, will always remain hidden. The dynamics presented here are reactions to danger to the inner essential self, sources of perceived danger such as ambiguity, and personal qualities.

Reactions to Danger

The anxious person's conscious inner world can allow them to function well in many parts of their lives. They are not in a highly anxious state all of the time and usually become so in response to real, or feared, or fantasized danger to the essential inner self. They do not assess the validity of the danger very well and can often respond to it as if it were at the highest level. All of the dangers referred to are possibilities of attack and/or destruction of their inner essential self. Their very being is under siege from external forces, and they doubt their competence to repel these attacks or to prevent the essential inner self from destruction. Their inability to assess the validity of the perceived danger, whether real or fantasized, is one reason that they feel the need to have others reassure them.

The anxious people described here also tend to perceive danger indiscriminately. This means that they can allow themselves to become agitated because they don't have all of the facts, cannot always know what someone else is thinking, are unable to completely and consistently control others or to control their environment, and are quick to fear and ascribe the worst to almost everything and everyone. They are very alert to any hint or possibility of perceived danger, and, when their alert system is triggered, they act on their anxiety and worry, micromanage, nag, or complain.

There is also the role for fantasized danger to their essential inner self, fantasized in the sense that there is no objective evidence of a possible attack on their self, or when what is feared is examined logically and rationally, is unlikely, is not possible, or is not realistic. Think of their fantasies as the flip side of the fantasy about winning millions of dollars in the lottery jackpot or some other major positive happening. These positive fantasies are great to contemplate but are very unlikely to happen for most of us. There may be some extremely slight chance that what they fear will happen but not very likely. This is one reason that the suggested responses in earlier chapters provided a procedure for threat assessment.

Reflection: Try to recall the underlying theme of most of the problems or concerns that your anxious person tends to bring to you most often and identify that theme in one or two words and if that theme is about a danger to their inner essential self. Examples of dangers can be that they will be perceived as inadequate, ineffective, wrong or shameful, or unworthy. This may help you understand the underlying triggers for their anxiety that sometimes seems over the top as a response to what is happening in the real world.

Sources of Perceived Danger

While it may seem that anything and everything is perceived by your anxious person as being dangerous for their essential inner self, the usual sources can be narrowed to two concepts: ambiguity and uncertainty. That is, the situation is ambiguous, and they are uncertain about their adequacy and competence. The external source or circumstance is not clear enough, and nothing will ever be clear enough for the anxious person as there are always intangibles; there are numerous and complex variables, all of which are not known to the person, and unanticipated events that can be contributing factors to the situation producing their anxiety. Everyone is faced with ambiguity every day in their lives, and many are able to navigate those adequately depending on their perception of their self-efficacy, their self-esteem, and the extent of their self-confidence. However, it is not so much that there is ambiguity; it is more of how the person feels about their ability to cope and manage with the needs and demands of the ambiguous situations, whether major or minor.

However, your anxious person cannot be comfortable with ambiguity and uncertainty and has a strong desire to know precisely what to expect, what they will need to do, and how to do what is needed for the situation. They want this knowledge beforehand and for every situation for fear of making mistakes, even minor ones that are of no consequence, or of appearing or feeling inadequate.

The other source of perceived danger comes from within the person. They do not feel adequate, competent, effective, or confident in their ability to survive. The many unknowns in ambiguity and uncertainty terrify them to a greater extent than for many others. This is terrifying for them because they cannot predict or control these unknowns. It doesn't help them to know that no one can predict or control unknowns or that others too may be uncomfortable with ambiguity and uncertainty. Their basic fear is the destruction of their essential inner self. They stay on alert almost all of the time but are especially alert when faced with ambiguity and uncertainty. Self-statement like the following may emerge for these anxious people:

I don't know what to do, and I'll make a mistake that will be devastating to me.

I must control others and/or the situation so that I will survive.

I have to win (be thought of as superior), or I will be ashamed.

Others are out to get me, and I need to protect myself.

As you can see, all of these self-statements seem to assume that there is danger and the self may not be adequate to forestall or combat the feared danger. Thus, fears fuel their anxiety.

Reflection: Do the self-statements seem to fit your anxious person? Is this especially true for ambiguous and uncertain situation that they face, and they seem to have many of these? While sometimes it is possible to prevent or anticipate what will be dangerous, this is not usually true for ambiguous and uncertain situations. Not only is the extent of the danger potentially destructive, but you don't know from whence the danger will come, how it will manifest itself, and if or when you will be destroyed. The anxious person in your life can not only experience this, but is not confident about their ability to survive which adds to their anxiety.

Life Experiences

Your anxious person does not always act out of fears of personal adequacy or fantasies; there can be a realistic component for their anxiety based on their past life experiences, especially those where they were chastised or blamed or shamed. Did you ever experience any of the following?

Told that you should be ashamed of yourself.

Blamed when something went wrong that was not your fault.

Had a parent or other adult tell you that you did something that made them ashamed of you, or that they did not want to be associated with you, or something similar.

Chastised for not being more like a sibling or someone else.

Felt guilty for disappointing a parent or other significant adult in your life.

Admonished for how you felt about something and told that you should not feel as you did.

Hopefully, if you could answer yes to any of these, it was an isolated event. Just think of what it would feel like to experience many of the examples and to experience those frequently over time. That is very corrosive and eroding to your self-confidence, self-efficacy, and self-esteem.

The anxious person in your life may be trying to ward off having to deal with the lingering feelings of being blamed or chastised as they were previously and their way of managing this is to worry, micromanage, nag, and/or complain. It could be that they are unconsciously still trying to please a parent, anticipate a parent's need or desire or wish so as to not be blamed for something not under their control, be seeking admiration and approval, and/or to prevent being shamed. While their current behavior and anxiety may be in response to a real-life situation, their past life experiences can also be an underlying contributor.

Reflection: Recall how you felt when you were blamed or chastised for something that you either did not do or were powerless to prevent. You don't carry this around with you all of the time, nor do you automatically go back to those feelings. Think of how you would probably feel if going back to the feelings aroused when unfairly blamed or chastised and this was your automatic response. That is what could happen for your anxious person.

Faulty Assumptions

Several faulty assumptions were presented in earlier chapters: limits of personal responsibility for others' welfare, a need for perfection in almost everything, and that making mistakes and errors is shameful. Other faulty assumptions can be similar to the following:

Everything will fall apart if I don't take care of it.

I cannot survive if others (anyone) disapproves of me.

I am adequate only when others agree that I am.

Compliments for others mean that I'm right, or better than adequate, or approved of and liked.

It's a catastrophe when things don't go as planned.

I should not make mistakes or errors.

Others should have the same commitment and obligations that I do.

Others should always recognize when things are wrong or need fixing and take care of it.

I do things correctly, and others should follow my example and not need reminding.

The way I want things done or demand that they be done is the "right" way.

Faulty assumptions can underlie behaviors, attitudes, and beliefs about oneself and about others and fuel the actions characterized as anxious. Faulty assumptions are unconscious and deeply held perceptions that are only partially or at times for the most part valid, but are usually invalid. I qualified some as partially valid because, under some circumstances, these assumptions or a particular assumption can be reasonable and valid to have. For example, operating surgeons should not make mistakes when operating. However, most of the listed assumptions are not usually valid and could be contributors to the inadequate self-perceptions the anxious person in your life may have.

Suggestion: Recall these faulty assumptions as you read Chapter 7 about the self-absorbed. Many of these are self-statements, even if false, as a part of self-absorption.

Tendencies

The anxious person in your life is likely to have several of the following tendencies. These are called tendencies because they are not all inclusive, meaning that the person does or exhibits this behavior, attitude, or reaction all of the time but they do most times. So it is called a tendency, not a characteristic. As you read the following tendencies, reflect on the extent to which each one fits the anxious person in your life.

Exaggerates the possibility of a catastrophe

Has unrealistic expectations of self and others

Pessimistic

Seeks (demands) perfection in self and others

Is unable to be gracious

Does not adjust to sudden changes

Overreacts to perceived criticism

Has to be "right"

Demands order, predictability, and consistency

Even when planned and orderly, does not manage transitions well

Personalizes others' comments, remarks, and so on.

Can be critical, demanding, and entitled

These tendencies can lead to internal distress, which then compels them to worry, micromanage, complain, and nag.

Reflection: Take some time to reflect on these as they could apply to you as well as to your anxious person. Think of how these tendencies could lead to being overly anxious, and most are unrealistic expectations of oneself.

Exaggerates the Possibility of Catastrophe

On some level the anxious person may know that the possibility of catastrophe is small or limited, but their definition of a catastrophe is broad and all encompassing. For example, most mistakes in everyday life do not lead to catastrophes. I am not considering major mistakes that lead to destruction of life and/or property. I am thinking of the common mistakes that are part of everyday life, are easily correctable in many instances, and are not life-threatening. However, for many of these anxious people, the possibility of making a mistake threatens their self-perception and self-esteem, hence they do fear that they will be destroyed for making a mistake. They work hard to prevent mistakes and fear that they will be blamed for mistakes that others make. This fear leads them to worry about remote possibilities for producing mistakes, micromanage others for fear that they will make mistakes, complain about mistakes or their possibility of appearing, and nag so that a possible mistake is prevented. Every mistake to them feels as if there will be dire consequences.

Has Unrealistic Expectations of Self and Others

Some anxiety emerges from the expectations we have of ourselves, and we strive to live up to our expectations such as acting in accord with our values. Realistic expectations for oneself are affirming and personally rewarding. However, when expectations for oneself are unrealistic and, these are also extended to encompass what is expected of others, that is where difficulties can emerge.

Let's continue to use the example of making mistakes to explain an unrealistic expectation. Even if you were to ask the anxious person in your life how realistic it is to expect to never make mistakes, you would not get a complete answer. Intellectually they would agree that it is unrealistic to expect that they would never make a mistake. On the emotional level, however, they are likely to feel that making a mistake is unforgiveable and that they are not worthy if they make a mistake, and to extend these feelings to also be about others. It is this emotional response that fuels their actions and unrealistic expectations.

There are many other unrealistic expectations they can have such as some of the following:

Always do your best

Always "win" or never lose or come in second

My perspective is "right"; others are "wrong"

Make sure that others never feel distress even when they can take care of themselves

Ensure that everything always goes as planned

Anticipate every potential glitch, problem, or barrier

Stay hypervigilant

Because they have these and/or other unrealistic thoughts and actions about themselves, they also tend to have the same expectations for others and can be deeply disappointed or even offended when others fail to meet the expectation(s). Anticipations of disappointment by oneself or by others can produce considerable anxiety.

Demanding Perfection

By far the most unrealistic expectation for the anxious person and/or for others is that of perfection. Striving for perfection can be a worthy goal and one to be pursued. However, when the goal of perfection is all encompassing and less than perfection for anything cannot be acceptable, then that unattainable goal becomes a liability. The anxious person can find that their functioning, self-esteem, self-efficacy, self-confidence, and relationships are negatively affected as their drive and demand for perfection affects many parts of their lives.

An expectation and demand for perfection is appropriate and understandable for many professions and tasks, and less-than-perfect could be life threatening in some instances. Unless your anxious person is trying to meet those standards where lives may be at risk, then their demands for perfection are excessive and can cause them and others considerable distress.

The anxious person in your life who can have an expectation of perfection can usually work hard to achieve that, but the problem is usually that they fret about it, obsess over minor and trivial details, expect others to be ready and willing to do what they are told to do at any time, and have other such thoughts, attitudes, and feelings but do not do any of this in isolation. They have to keep you informed of every fleeting thought, possibility, and the like along the way. Yes, you know just how anxious they are and how much it means to them to be perfect always and for everything. They cause themselves and others considerable distress in their efforts to attain perfection.

Many adults learn somewhere in the journey to adulthood that good enough can be acceptable for some things, at some times, and under some circumstances, and do not blame themselves for not being perfect all of the time. However, your anxious person most likely did not internalize that acceptance and, as an adult, continue to blame themselves and others for everything that is less than perfect.

Unable to Be Gracious

Your anxious person may find it difficult or even impossible to be gracious in the sense of being kind and forgiving of mistakes, errors, lapses in judgment, and so on. They do not accept and may not forgive these in themselves, nor can they do so for others. They are harsh on themselves and on others.

Let's look at a few examples of lack of graciousness:

A teen who was usually reliable but forgot that he was supposed to cut the grass and was chastised and punished

A subordinate called on the carpet because she did not get the information the boss wanted because of unforeseen circumstances where the person who had the information had a medical emergency

A spouse who picked out a gift in a disliked color and was told to exchange it

The parent who did not post the picture a child drew because it did not fit the color scheme

Some anxious people are so desirous of perfection that they fail to account for human lapses, or misunderstandings, or even errors. Some things that many others can forgive, overlook, or be accepting of, they cannot. They may be able to hide their true feelings at times, but then they still have some resentment that the other person was not correct, right, or perfect. They tend to operate on the basis of should and ought.

Sudden Changes

These anxious people do not adjust to sudden changes very well, and their anxiety can intensify to unmanageable levels when faced with something immediate, unexpected, and unanticipated. While many of us may also have our anxiety elevated under these circumstances, it is not to the level that theirs gets. The least little change in almost anything seems to get them off-balance, confused, and even panicky.

It is very comforting and pleasurable to know what to expect and these expectations are met. Tasks are completed well and in a timely manner, problems are few and any that exist are minor and easily taken care of, and matters seem to go as planned. We can all enjoy and appreciate those times when things go well, or even mostly so. What may be difficult for us to imagine is that the anxious person may never or seldom experience this as their fears and apprehensions keep them in a constant state of pre-paring for fight or flight, and, although they may be anticipating some-thing dire, they are not prepared for or able to cope with sudden changes, glitches, and other such events. For example, a Micromanager may not have an alternative in mind if a key person were to become ill or there is a crisis where they are not available.

Sudden changes may arouse extreme anxiety for the anxious person in your life because they are already insecure about their adequacy and are not able to do anything but react in the moment as if their inner essential self were in danger of being destroyed. They are concerned that others will be able to see their inadequacy, incompetency, and inability to cope, and this is very shaming. They may also think that what they fear about themselves has validity, and this is extremely shaming and troubling for them. They try to hide these thoughts, concerns, and feelings by express-ing intense anxiety about the change or glitch, but the underlying con-cern is about their core essential inner self.

Cannot Tolerate Criticism

The anxious person in your life may be hypersensitive to any hint of perceived criticisms. While the anxious person can be very self-critical or oblivious to any faults that others see, they do not tolerate any suggestion from others that they are in error, made a mistake, misunderstood, or are inadequate in any way. The other person does not have to directly criti-cize or even intend to be critical, but the anxious person receives it as critical. It may even be that the absence of a comment or remark is taken as being critical of them.

Criticism is very wounding to the anxious person as this can highlight for them their imperfection. No matter their words that acknowledge an intellectual understanding that perfection is aspirational and unattain-able, their core belief is that they must be perfect in order to survive.

Thus, when others see and remark on imperfections, they become wounded and fearful, which can help explain some of their reactions to intended or unintended criticism. What some others are able to shrug off or take in as being constructive feedback, they cannot.

Has to Be "Right"

It does not seem to make a difference what the topic is, the anxious person has to be "right" all of the time and about everything. The matter may be trivial for others, but it is essential to that person that they are "right" even in the face of facts or other evidence of other perspectives. Their way is the "right" way to do almost anything, and others would do well to follow their lead.

Just as with other described behaviors, attitudes, and beliefs, being "right" is affirming that they are worthy and being "wrong" is shaming and wounding. They will argue, insist, demand, and otherwise act to get others to agree that they are "right." The flip side is that they are also insistent that others are "wrong" and have to admit it. They assume that others feel as they do, that being wrong is shaming. This can be one reason that they insist on being acknowledged as being "right" because that also acknowledges that others are "wrong" and hence are shameful. They can then boast their self-perception and self-esteem about being superior because they are "right."

Order, Predictability, and Control

Central to the anxious person's worldview is their need for order, predictability, and control, and these are what they seek to relieve their anxiety. Although their fears are about their essential inner self, they are able to look to the external world to provide them with the means to affirm and support their essential inner self, and when there is order, predictability, and control, they can feel safe that their essential inner self is capable and adequate and that they will be able to survive.

If you reflect on the matters or events that produce distress for the anxious person in your life, you will probably find that what they verbalize can be summed up as a lack of order, or a lack of predictability, or a lack of control. They are not so different from most everyone else in this, but where they do differ is in the intensity of the feelings that are aroused, and their resulting actions.

These anxious people can value order to the point where they demand that others conform to their idea of what order is and should be.

Examples can include how the dishwasher is loaded, how your clothes should be placed in drawers, the sequence for getting dressed, and other such activities. Their need for predictability can be seen in how they cannot adjust to minor setbacks such as a traffic jam where they have to take an alternate route, calling someone who is usually there but that day they are not, or expecting something that does not materialize. They can continually seek control over others, events, and situations where they could expect to have little or no control, which causes them to be uneasy and seek even more control over people and events in their lives where they may have some control.

Trying to improve order, predictability, and control can be very frustrating, and the results are usually not as favorable as would be desired. However, the anxious person's inner world seems to compel them to try and do so even in the face of continual failure. Their needs and attempts to meet these keep them in a constant state of agitation and stress.

The anxious person in your life is likely not to manage transitions well. Transitions as used here refer to anticipated or planned changes. Unlike unanticipated events, these are known in advance and the changes can be managed to be as least disruptive as possible.

When I say that they do not manage transitions well, I mean that they become even more worried, micromanaging, and complaining than they usually are. Even the most orderly and planned transition produces intense anxiety that they find difficult to contain and manage. They can fret about inconsequential matters, become compulsive about checking and rechecking, seek to impose order and control in almost every part of their lives, and need almost constant reassurance. Transitions for many of us can be unsettling and disruptive even those for which we planned and may even desire. There is a lot of ambiguity and uncertainty around transitions, and it would not be unusual for us to experience some apprehension about the change and our ability to cope. All of these reactions can be expected. What differs for the anxious person is that their reactions are more intense and negative, and they look to others for relief, reassurance, and comfort even more often than usual.

It is not so much that there is a transition since these happen throughout life and some are desirable and pleasurable; it is more that the anxious person in your life seems to need you more and that can take a toll on your and on the relationship. It's not as if your life stopped and you don't have personal matters and concerns so that all you have to do is to take care of the anxious person in your life. You now have to manage both your life and their continual and constant anxiety during the transition.

Personalizes Almost Everything

Whether directed at them or not, the anxious person in your life may tend to personalize most everything. They can think that the comment, remark, or action was intended to be dismissive, blaming, critical, and/or shaming of them, sometimes even when others are named. They see others' words and actions as that person's way of saying that they are not good enough. What actually occurs many times is that their negative feelings about themselves are triggered by what someone else says or does and they automatically think that the person means them. These negative feelings about oneself can be triggered when they feel

Ignored—not attended to in a positive way

Dismissed—as being not important enough

Devalued—as not being worthy of attention or mention

Diminished—not perceived to us as good as others

Inadequate—not good enough

Criticized—not good enough

Blamed—wrong, shameful

Their sense of their essential inner self as being fatally flawed allows these negative thoughts and feelings about their selves to be triggered at any time and by many things or people in their lives. Some can think that no matter what or who someone is talking about, their real target is them.

Can Be Critical, Demanding, and Feel Entitled

On the other hand, the anxious person in your life may tend to be critical, demanding, and have an entitlement attitude. They can be critical of others for not being good enough, making mistakes, or being perfect. They can be demanding of others to conform to what they want or need them to be or do; that others attend to their needs, wishes, and desires; and that others be admiring of them. They can have an entitlement attitude that dismisses as invalid any criticism and allows them to put their needs, wishes, or desires as priorities for others, to be critical of others, and to receive preferential treatment all or almost all of the time.

Reflect back to the description of the anxious person's inner world to get some idea of why they are so critical and demanding and have an entitlement attitude. They are constantly battling internal chaos as well as the fear of not being adequate or good enough. In addition, some of these anxious people cannot or do not clearly and sufficiently differentiate themselves from others (poor boundaries), which can cause them to perceive others as extensions of themselves and others are thereby under their control.

So when the world doesn't seem to be orderly, predictable, or controllable, and others are not rushing in to see to it that their world is as they think it should be, this arouses their anxiety, which fuels their criticism and demands because they feel entitled to have their world as they want it to be.

Some anxious people can feel entitled to

Criticize and blame you for not ensuring their comfort and well-being (reducing or eliminating their inner chaos)

Give orders and expect prompt compliance

Intrude on you when they are anxious and want something from you

Expect you to be available when needed

Have their needs and demands as your priority

Request or demand favors with no reciprocity

Have you and others admire them

Receive preferential treatment from everyone or almost everyone, and almost all of the time

Many of these anxious people are not aware of their entitlement attitude and would be very offended if you pointed it out. But some of their conscious actions and thoughts are manifestations of their entitlement attitude.

Withholds Approval

It may be that the anxious person is so caught up in their current experiencing that they do not have the time or energy to be aware of their impact on others, or they are indifferent to others when in this state, or for some other reasons, they are discounting how others may be reacting to them. The next section in this chapter goes into more detail about some self-absorbed behaviors and attitudes your anxious person may display. However, the topic at this point is on withholding approval, which may not be a conscious act, but does or can affect their relationships.

Just think about it. Does the anxious person in your life verbalize approval of anything or only does so infrequently? Do you recall the Micromanager voicing approval of what has been done or how well it was done? Does the Complainer notice when something is acceptable or only when something is unacceptable? Can you think of any time when the Nagger noticed that you met expectations? Or, when the Worrier talked about what was going right for them? Whereas they seem to want approval and appreciation for their attending to matters or preventing potential problems, or ensuring order and control, or for correcting what doesn't meet expectations, they do not seem to notice or approve when things do go right. Indeed, some of these anxious people do not seem to approve of anything, or, at least, they do not voice this approval.

It is very likely that these anxious people are so focused on their inner chaos that they cannot attend to others especially when they are agitated. They may also stay in a state where they feel that they must be alert to potential problems and the like and are so focused on the negatives that they do not have any time and energy to notice the positives, which can be troubling and erode their immediate relationships.

What They Cannot See

Although this section is titled "What They Cannot See," what follows also applies to everyone. We all have a part of ourselves that we cannot see. I like to use the analogy of trying to see the back of your head without the use of a mirror, which cannot be done. However, other people can see the back of our heads, and that analogy is what is proposed here that you and others can see parts of the anxious person that they cannot see. It may be difficult to accept but has lots of validity, that others can see parts of ourselves that we cannot see. The following activity may help illustrate what is meant.

The Hidden Self

Materials—four to five sheets of paper, a writing instrument (a part of the activity that will ask you to spread out the sheets side by side, which could be difficult or impossible to implement on a computer or tablet, which is the rationale for not suggesting the use of electronic devices), and a suitable surface for writing.

Procedure:

1. Gather materials and find a place to work where you will not be disturbed.
2. Use the first sheet of paper and title it "Open Parts of Self" to make a list of those topics about yourself that you can readily disclose to others whom you

do not know well. These can be parts such as occupation, country or region of origin, favorite reading material or TV shows, and the like.

3. Use the next sheet of paper and title it "Open to Family and Close Friends." Make a list of those aspects of yourself that you readily disclose to many if not all of family and close friends: aspects such as your aspirations, hopes, dreams, plans, and the like.

4. Take another sheet of paper and title it "My Secrets" to make a list of those parts of yourself that you are aware of but do not disclose to others. Items such as impossible dreams and wishes, longing, regrets, likes, and dislikes. You can use words, phrases, or symbols to represent these if you like.

5. Use another sheet of paper and title it "Others See Me." List what others see about you that you do not see including characteristics that you do not agree with, criticisms (these do not have to be accurate), and anything you think might fit here. An item on this list does not need to have several people commenting on it, but be sure to list actions, attitudes, and beliefs others have noted about you.

6. Take the final sheet of paper and title it "Hidden Aspects of Myself." This will be the hardest list to construct because these are beliefs, attitudes, feelings, and the like that you are not aware of or have repressed and denied them. Following are some possibilities:

    Self-absorbed behaviors and attitudes (a full list is provided in Chapter 7), such as attention and admiration needs

    Shameful thoughts, attitudes, and/or behaviors

    Vanity

    Pride

    Envy and jealousy

    A fighting spirit, hardiness, and/or resilience

    Inspirers

    Creativity

    Longings and yearnings

    Determination

    Notice that there can be some positive characteristics, and these are some unrecognized and unused inner resources that can be helpful.

7. Spread out the five lists side by side from 1 to 5. Review what you listed and add items to a list or move items to another list. Try not to delete any items you first listed.

8. Reflect on your layers to see if you are appropriately revealing parts of yourself or if some parts are revealed to inappropriate audiences. For example, it may not be appropriate to reveal guilt to casual acquaintances. Also, reflect on if you are keeping aspects of yourself hidden that could be enriching to a

relationship such as with an intimate partner. Finally, look at the "Others See Me" list and reflect on how the items could be valid including criticisms. You may want to try and reflect on what behaviors or attitudes could have led to the comment or criticism.

Now that you have worked through the activity for yourself, you may be better able to understand why the anxious person in your life cannot see what or how they are contributing to their own anxiety.

A Role of Self-absorption

A very important aspect of oneself that is hidden or mostly hidden is the level and extent of one's self-absorption as an adult. Self-absorption for adults is used here to describe the behaviors and attitudes that reflect an undeveloped psychological part of self. Undeveloped means that the behaviors and attitudes exhibited are more like those that would be expected and seen in a child. For example, it is expected that a child would exhibit actions similar to the following.

- Grandiosity–Saying and believing, "I can do anything"
- Entitlement–The 2-year-old who has a tantrum for not immediately receiving what is wanted or demanded
- Attention-seeking–The child who acts in accord with "Look at me, look at me now!"
- Extensions of self–Not recognizing others' personal boundaries or possessions

Some of these behaviors may be endearing when exhibited by a child, but are troubling and off-putting for adult behavior and attitudes. The next chapter describes the self-absorbed behaviors and attitudes that may have a role in the behaviors and attitudes of the anxious person in your life, could be negatively impacting their relationships and may be fueling some of their anxiety.

CHAPTER SEVEN

Anxious and Self-absorbed

There are some self-absorbed behaviors and attitudes the anxious person in your life may exhibit. One important point to remember as you read these descriptions is that your anxious person cannot see these behaviors and attitudes as reflective of self-absorption or can deny that they do any of these. My recommendation is that you read these descriptions for a better understanding of the anxious person in your life and not try to tell them about any of their behaviors and attitudes that may be self-absorbed as this is unlikely to be received positively. As you read these, reflect on how or if these fit for the Worrier, the Complainer, the Micromanager, and the Nagger.

Described are the following some characteristics of self-absorption they may exhibit often or almost always.

- Has an overly inflated self-perception
- Acts on the basis of a deflated self-perception
- Demonstrates an entitlement attitude
- Thrives on receiving attention, for example, being needier than others, or as being more superior
- Seeks excessive praise and admiration
- Does not recognize or respect others' personal boundaries
- Takes advantage of others' willingness to help them
- Verbalizes that others get breaks that they do not get but which they deserve
- Seldom if ever empathizes with you or others
- Perceives others as happy and they are not
- Stunted emotional experiencing and expressions

An Overly Inflated Self-perception

An overly inflated self-perception carries the unconscious or conscious assumption that one is grand, all knowing, superior, without flaws or faults, able to do anything and everything excellently, and that others should recognize how they are better. Some examples that may help describe behaviors and attitudes that can indicate an overly inflated sense of oneself are similar to the following:

A tendency to overcommit and take on too many tasks at one time and then feeling overwhelmed and stressed

Not being prepared adequately and expecting a pass or having a ready excuse

Agree to assume responsibility for something without first assuring that they will have the time or expertise for the task

Assuming that their perspective or viewpoint is more valid than are others, and denigrating any perspective that is not in agreement with theirs

Have a conviction that they have the "right" answers for just about everything

Knowing which is "right" for others and what they should or ought to be or do

Tending to act in an arrogant manner, especially when they feel challenged

There are many other everyday examples. The anxious person in your life may display some of these behaviors and attitudes.

Reflection: Make a note of each overly inflated self-perception your anxious person seems to display frequently.

A Deflated Self-perception

A deflated self-perception is the flip side of the overly inflated self-perception, and both self-perceptions co-exist within the same person. That is, the deflated self exists in tandem with the inflated self but may be exhibited at different times and with different people. But, first, let's describe the deflated self-perception and how this may be seen in the behaviors and attitudes of anxious person in your life.

- A "poor me" demeanor.
- Frequently expressing helplessness or even hopelessness.
- Feeling that they are picked on or dismissed or irrelevant.
- "The sky is falling" perspective about many things. Seems to always expect a catastrophe.
- "Woe is me, what should I do" seems to be a mantra.

- May frequently say that they can't catch a break.
- Expresses that others are more (successful, adequate, capable) than they are.
- Feels that they do not get (respect, or appreciation).

There are numerous ways in which an impoverished ego may be found.

However, the flip side is the inflated self, which was noted as coexisting with the deflated self, and an interesting thing is that this can flip-flop quickly in interactions so that when you respond to one, such as the deflated self, the person's response illustrates their overly inflated self. Suppose that you are interacting with your anxious person who has come to you with a concern because they can't see how to handle it, and you try to give a helpful solution, only to have them say that they can take care of the concern and don't need advice. This can be very confusing because they come to you in the deflated state, you respond to it, but their comment to your response is from the inflated self.

Reflection: List the most frequent behaviors that indicate a deflated self-state that your anxious person exhibits.

An Entitlement Attitude

The behaviors associated with this attitude can be hard to pinpoint in the moment, or many are identified in retrospect after some thought is given. The entitlement attitude seems to be one that elevates the person above others and protects them from having to suffer the consequences of their actions, have an unspoken expectation that others are aware of their importance and that they must and should receive preferential treatment, and that rules (laws and the like) should not and do not apply to them. Examples for an entitlement attitude include the following:

- An expectation that their needs and wants will be attended to without their asking or saying anything.
- Not being punished for rule infractions.
- Taking the possessions of others without their permission.
- Saying what comes to mind that is rude without any consideration for the impact it may have on other person.
- Interrupting when others are talking.
- Demanding attention or that they must get whatever they want.
- Their needs, wants, or desires receive your priority attention.
- Expecting prompt obedience to their demands.

- Warnings, cautious, and the like don't apply to them, such as doing risky things even after being warned.
- Intruding on and disrupting others for what they consider to be important.
- Making a scene if they don't get their way.
- Calling people distasteful names or detracting labels.

While most of these actions can be expected of children, when they are done by adults, they are not enchanting, excusable, or easily dismissed. It's as if the person feels that they can do whatever they want to, and others should just accept it. In addition, they seem to think that others should recognize their superiority without question. These are some of the more extreme examples for the entitlement attitude in adults.

However, there are also some milder everyday actions that many adults do that can suggest an entitlement attitude. Do any of these fit the anxious person or you?

- Exceed the speed limit
- Push to the front of a line
- Make remarks that are put-downs, dismissive, and/or devaluing of others
- Fail to acknowledge or show appreciation for what someone does for them
- Engage in risky behavior(s) without thoughts or consideration for negative consequences
- Tell people what they should or ought to do as you perceive it without being asked
- Become angry or annoyed when you do not receive preferential treatment
- Think that their welfare and well-being should be a priority for others
- Give orders and expect prompt obedience

These actions can be unconscious assumptions that accompany an entitlement attitude. The person, on some level, perceives themselves as having the right or entitled to ignore rules, or policies as laws; put others in their inferior places; to do and say what they want; and/or have their well-being as others' priorities.

Reflection: List all of the behaviors that your anxious person frequently exhibits, and add others that seem to you to be reflective of an entitlement attitude.

Thrives on Receiving Attention

There is a whole industry around seeking and getting attention and some occupations and demand the spotlight and attention such as performers on stage, TV, and in films; politicians; and writers. Attention is important for their survival and promotion. However, the attention-seeking behavior referred to here is not a part of someone's professional life or well-being; it's just a part of what the person does and says in the effort to ensure that they are always or almost always the center of attention. Some of the following may fit the anxious person in your life:

- Talks loudly and talks a lot
- Makes provocative comments so that others ask for more information
- Carps, kvetches, and complains very often
- Boasts and brags about possessions, achievements, or even their children
- Plays "Can you top this!" and other such games
- Interrupts and intrudes into other people's conversation
- Has to have the last word on almost everything
- Dresses and/or acts to bring attention to them
- Sulks in a way to ensure that others notice
- Loudly points out other's mistakes, flaws, and the like in the presence of others
- Chastises someone when others are present
- Most always engages in one-upmanship
- Tells jokes and funny stories, some of which are inappropriate
- Pokes fun at others' inadequacies, flaws, and/or deficiencies

Some attention at sometimes can be welcome, and it can be affirming to be noticed and appreciated. However, when the person's actions are always or almost always designed to get and keep them in the spotlight or as the focus of attention, that can indicate some self-absorption.

Reflection: List the actions of your anxious person that are descriptive of a need for attention. Also try to describe how they behave when the wanted attention is not forthcoming.

Seeks Excessive Praise and Admiration

I don't know of anyone who doesn't want to be appreciated, valued, and recognized by others. It is very affirming of one's efforts, of our accomplishments, and to know that others find us to be worthwhile and admirable in some way. Yes, we are pleased when we receive compliments, others' approval, and even awards. Being admiration needy drives the person's behavior to seek reassurance that they are superior to others, more valued, and worthwhile, and that they should receive more exten-sive recognition of these.

Some admiration-needy behaviors and attitudes include the following. As you read these, reflect on the extent to which your anxious person exhibits these, or if you tend to do them.

- Feel that they suffer more than most everyone else, and ensures that others are aware of the extent to which they suffer
- Stay in a bad or destructive relationship or situation when there are other options and lets others know just how bad everything is for them
- Constantly fish for compliments and other affirmations and approvals
- Continually apply for awards or have someone nominate them for recognitions and awards
- Boast and brag
- Exaggerate accomplishments, prominent contacts, personal characteristics considered as positive, salary, and so on.
- Status seeking such as joining certain clubs, only or mostly associating with certain people and the like
- Must have the approval of almost everyone in order to feel adequate.
- Can convey an attitude of self-satisfaction.

The anxious person in your life may display some of the admiration-needy behaviors and attitudes. For example, the Micromanager may be excessive in their attention to details and ensure that the task is prop-erly completed and also wants to be appreciated for their efforts. The Complainer may be seeking approval for noticing what is not correct or needs to be done and verbalizing this so that action can be taken to correct it.

Reflection: Try to describe the lengths to which your anxious person goes to get admiration. How important does this seem to be for them?

Does Not Recognize or Respect Others' Boundaries

This concept is not easy to describe as it refers to an internal percep-tion of the unseen demonstration of where you end and where others begin. Some of the behaviors and attitudes described that are sugges-tive of an incomplete perception and understanding of where you end and where others begin can contribute to extensions of self as an indi-cator of an excessive self-focus. Some examples include actions like the following:

Engages in unexpected or unwanted and/or unwelcome intrusions or interruptions

Invades your and others' personal space such as standing too close, gives you uninvited touching or hugging, or enters your room or office without waiting for an invitation

Takes or uses your possessions without asking or waiting for permission

Assumes that others have the same feelings or perceptions that they do

Has a conviction or mind-set that others, including children, should have the same values or attitudes and the like as they do in order to be accepted and worthwhile

Speaks for others such as for a spouse or partner.

Tells others what they should or ought to do or think or be

Gives orders or demands and expects prompt compliance or obedience

Has a perception that others are under their control and should do what they want them to do.

Has an expectation that others should "know," that is, read their mind, what is needed or wanted, and provide this without having to be asked and anticipate and fulfill their desires, wants, and needs.

The anxious person in your life who has an incomplete understanding of where they end and where others begin can be oblivious to when they are violating or intruding on your boundaries. They do things such as calling you at all hour, interrupting you when they feel a need to take care of their anxiety regardless of what you are doing, demanding that you attend promptly to their agenda and make that your priority, assuming that you think or have the same opinions as that they do, standing too close or touch without asking permission, chastising or blaming you for not doing what they think you "ought to know to do without their having to tell you," and many other acts that are suggestions that they are not aware or respectful of your psychological boundaries.

Reflection: Write a short paragraph that captures the behaviors and attitudes of the anxious person in your life that suggest lack of understanding about their and others' boundaries.

Takes Unfair Advantage of Others' Willingness to Help

Using people to attain personal gains is our definition for taking advantage or exploitation. "Using" in this definition refers to taking unfair advantage, seduction, misleading, capitalizing on their good nature or ignorance, or any other such actions that result in personal gains at the expense of someone else. Think about the following as examples of exploitation:

- Asking for or demanding favors with no reciprocity
- Requesting others to do something that they you could do for themselves
- Stealing or co-opting others' ideas
- Misleading others to give them something they want (think of scams and cons)
- Misusing a relationship to get something that they want or want the other person to do
- Misusing the power differential between them and the other person for personal favors or gain
- Borrowing possessions without asking permission
- Violating the trust that someone has in them
- Withholding information, resources, and the like to manipulate others into doing what they want them to do
- Engaging in power plays

There are numerous ways to engage in exploitive behavior, and some are done without conscious intent. For example, a parent doesn't intend to exploit a child by asking the child to do something the parent could do for themselves. Nor is a colleague necessarily intending to be exploitive by asking for a favor, but never seems to be in a place where they are able to return favors. Have you ever borrowed something like a book or tool and failed to return it? On the other hand, has a family member or friend asked you for a favor that caused you some time and effort or was inconvenient, but you did it anyway because you have difficulty saying no to the person and they know that you would have difficulty turning them down? All exploitation is not major, such as romantic seduction or a scam where someone can be hurt or suffer a significant loss, or intentionally exploitative, but the level and extent of the exploitation does not lessen its impact or outcome. Some of these behaviors are common everyday occurrences. The exploiter gains at the other person's expense.

Reflection: List the feelings that were triggered when reading this section on exploitation, and describe how you feel when you think the anxious person in your life is trying to or is exploiting you.

Feel More Deserving Than Others

It is common to experience some minor envy occasionally or infrequently, to wish for what someone else has or does. When envying becomes a regular reaction as happens frequently, this can indicate some troubling self-absorption because this level of envy assumes that others are less worthy or less deserving. In other words, the envied person should not have what is desired and the person who is envious should have it because they are more worthy or more deserving.

Envy seems to be a cry for recognition for superiority and can be about almost anything, the envied person's possessions, relationships, talent, accomplishments, recognitions such as awards or promotions, personal qualities such as contentment or determination, and so on. The envious person feels that they either do not have what the envied person has or that they do have it but is nothing recognized by others, and that they should have it or be recognized because they are superior. In some way the envious person can feel that they are being cheated out of something they deserve and are resentful.

It is this resentment and feeling of superiority that makes envy corrosive to one's self-esteem. Someone else got what was desired, and by doing so is receiving something unfairly that they do not warrant. The important point in the discussion is that envy is self-defeating because it takes time, energy, and effort away from more important things in the envious person's life. An example would be envying a promotion that someone received. Now, while it is understandable to also want or yearn for a promotion, it does not help to be resentful or envious of the other person, instead of determining what is needed for you to achieve the promotion and work toward that goal. Or, let's take envying someone who has talent that you do not have or have in a modest amount. What is more useful and affirming for you? To resent that person's talent or to work to develop that modest talent you do have? Or, to acknowledge and recognize your differing talent and capitalize on that? You will be better off building your talents, either working to acquire or saving to get the possessions you want and fostering the development of your inner resources and qualities.

The anxious person in your life may be unreasonably envious of others in their lives, which, as noted before, can be corrosive to their self-esteem. This erosion of their self-esteem can then help to produce worry, micromanaging, nagging, and complaining. If they felt they were good enough as others are or seem to be, they could prevent disaster for themselves and for others and ensure that tasks were properly completed, things are done right or as they should be, or everything was perfect with no complaints.

Reflection: Reflect on whether the anxious person in your life or if you tend to be envious.

A Poor Emotional Life

A capacity to experience deep and intense feelings such as love, grief, enthusiasm, or passionate commitment contributes to enriching life, relationships, and other meaningful connections in our lives. Some people's emotional life is very limited where their experiencing and expressions are few, and those few tend to be negative such as anger and fear. The other characteristic of their emotional lives is that they do linger in any emotion. A shallow emotional life can facilitate the lack of meaning and purpose for their lives, as well as a lack of meaningful and enduring relationships. They are able to hop from relationship to relationship without any ill effects on them.

They may also not understand why others feel as they do or continue to stay with a particular feeling because, after all, they get over their negative feelings rather quickly and easily. They may not understand why someone continues to be sad, glad, or apprehensive because they don't. Even when they express an emotion, there does not seem to be much substance to it. They can use the words, but they do not have the feeling that usually accompanies the word.

A shallow emotional life could be described as experiencing pale versions of rich emotions. For example:

Pleasure but not joy

Appreciation but not gratitude

Interest but not excitement

Pleased but not happy

Delight but not bliss

Comfort but not cheerfulness

This shallowness also includes the tendency to jump from emotion to emotion rather quickly. For example, the person may be annoyed or angry about something significant at one point, but, if you asked them later about the anger-provoking incident, they not only are no longer angry but they now term it as being of no consequence. While we can all appreciate the capacity to relinquish negative emotions, we usually do not discuss or minimize the provocation. The tendency is what allows them to easily and frequently move from relationship to relationship.

Reflection: Make a list of all of the feelings you had in the past two days, and put a checkmark by those that reoccur. How many different ones did you experience? How many of them were deep or intense? Are your emotions shallow? Does the anxious person in your life tend to have shallow emotions?

An Inability to Be Empathic

A major characteristic of self-absorption is a lack of empathy. Empathy is not catching others' feelings as described in earlier chapters as "catching" speaks to insufficient or poor psychological boundary strength. When someone is empathic, that person has some good and strong psychological boundary strength, can voluntarily feel what the other person is feeling, and is conscious of what they are doing.

Psychological boundary strength is a necessary component for empathy because it prevents you from becoming overwhelmed or enmeshed in the other person's feelings, helps you to sustain the perception of yourself as separate and distinct from the other person, and allows you to let go of the other person's feelings when you tuned into those. Empathy is voluntary in the sense that you make a conscious decision to open yourself and enter the world of the other to feel what that person is feeling. Catching is an involuntary and unconscious act because no decision is consciously made; the catching just happens. Chapters 2 and 3 explain this process and why you are susceptible to "catching" others' feelings, especially those broadcast by adults.

Lack of empathy may not be an all-or-nothing characteristic for some people. They may be somewhat capable of being empathic with some people some of the time, but that can be seldom. Nor am I suggesting that you should be empathic with everyone or almost everyone all of the time as that would be exhausting and just about impossible. What is possible and helpful is to be empathic with some people, such as the anxious person in your life, some of the time.

Lack of empathy in interactions can be illustrated by the following examples:

- An abrupt change of topic when talking with another person
- Introduction of a new topic to avoid the other person's emotional intensity
- Interjecting an off-topic response in an interaction
- Not listening to the speaker and thinking about personal or other things
- Failure to acknowledge the speaker's feelings
- Providing a response that ignores the speaker's feelings and focuses only on the content of the message
- Telling jokes and funny stories to get away from the speaker's emotional intensity
- Deflecting the conversation or interaction by bringing others into the conversation
- Using sarcasm as a response

These are just a few examples and you can probably think of other examples for when someone demonstrated a lack of empathy for you. Since the anxious person in your life is someone with whom you want to maintain a relationship, you want to be empathetic much of the time. However, there may be times when not focusing on their feelings could be helpful for whatever the current situation is. For example, if your anxious person is becoming mired in an intense emotion, you may want to just acknowledge their feeling but not empathize and feel it also.

Reflection: How empathic is your anxious person with you and with others? Do you find that when you are empathic with them you "catch" their feelings? Do you ever wish that you were not as empathic as you are? If so, that may signal that you tend to become enmeshed or overwhelmed by others' feelings.

An Inner Void

Nothing is very difficult to describe, and definitions usually define nothing as a void or absence, or as nothing, but those definitions are not very helpful especially when trying to describe the internal psychological concept of emptiness. Emptiness is not depression where there can be considerable deflation of the inner core self and suppressed and/or repressed feelings. The deflated essential inner core self is there as are the feelings that cannot be accessed. Emptiness at the core of oneself is different as there is nothing to be accessed, available, or helpful.

Let's try to explain core emptiness as an absence of some usually adult human understandings, awareness, and deeply held convictions. This adult has all or many of the following.

- An awareness and appreciation of others as separate and distinct from them.
- A set of core values that are adhered to, and that guide most of their actions.
- An understanding of how to initiate and maintain meaningful and enduring relationships.
- They accept and act on the premise that life has meaning and purpose and that this affirms and sustains their existence beyond the basics needed to survive.
- An understanding that relationships are to be cultivated and not exploited.
- An inner life that includes access to many and some intense emotions.
- A capacity to feel and express love, joy, and enthusiasm/zest.

The inner void termed "emptiness" has to be described in terms of something. This makes it almost impossible for most of us to actually contemplate and understand emptiness. There are some behaviors and attitudes that may signal that someone may be empty at the core.

- Few if any meaningful and enduring relationships.
- Shifting, changing, and insubstantial values as demonstrated by actions. No discernable consistency seems to underlie their decisions, affiliations, and/or actions.
- Lots of drama. Usually initiated in the effort to feel something, to manipulate and control others, or to demonstrate their power.
- An unending need, desire, and bid for attention and admiration from everyone or almost everyone.
- Excessive envy of others demonstrated by their denigration, dismissiveness, and/or minimizing of others.
- Inflating personal accomplishments, characteristics, actions, possessions, and the like.
- Engages in capricious actions, and will say one thing mean another, act in accordance with neither.

In contrast, people who are not empty at the core of their inner essential self are able to have and experience many or most of the characteristics listed earlier in this section as usual adult human understandings, awareness, and deeply held convictions.

Reflection: Would you characterize your anxious person as empty or as having an essential core self with meaning and purpose for their lives, being able to initiate and maintain meaningful relationships, and having other characteristics that show that they are not empty?

Inappropriate Humor

One major characteristic of some people's underdeveloped narcissism is inappropriate humor. Some may call it juvenile because of its insensitivity, callousness, and hurtful effects. Jokes, comments, stories, and remarks that are intended to be humorous put-downs or denigrations, in an attempt to shame, or to humiliate, or show how the target is inferior and that the speaker is superior, and other such intents and outcomes are examples of inappropriate humor. Especially egregious are comments and the like that focus on a person's characteristics about which they can do nothing to change such as a person's height, skin color, or disability.

Attention is being focused here on how supposedly humorous remarks and the like are really intended to be shaming for the target. Examples of this can be seen in comments that focus on the following.

Body image
Religion
Age and its effects
Political affiliation
Denigration of women
Socioeconomic status
Education and/or its lack
Sexual orientation

So-called taunting and teasing may be intended as humor by some, but the underlying intent and purpose are to humiliate and shame the other person and to show how they are inferior to the speaker. These are only some examples for inappropriate humor.

Reflection: How often does your anxious person use inappropriate humor? Do you sometimes wish that they would not taunt, tease, or make fun of others?

Is Your Anxious Person Also Very Self-absorbed?

After reading these descriptions, you may find that several of these fit the anxious person in your life. You may be tempted to try and make them aware of their troubling behaviors and attitudes in an effort to show them that they could be less anxious if they were less self-absorbed. However, the one thing you should not do is to confront them as you will then run into what I term as a "narcissistic wall." Confrontation does and will not work because they are unaware of what they are doing and seeing that you are terming as self-absorbed behavior or attitude. For example, they will not see themselves as having an entitlement attitude.

They Are Unaware

People who have considerable self-absorption may not be diagnosed as having a Narcissistic Personality Disorder (NPD) but can still display and have some of those same behaviors and attitudes although theirs may be fewer and less intense. In addition, other people who interact with them frequently may not realize the extent of self-absorption and what this can mean for how they relate and communicate. This unawareness usually produces frustration, self-doubt, hurt, and even rage in others who interact with them on a regular basis. The self-absorbed person's relating and communication style can trigger these feelings in you and others who may then try to use confrontation as a way to make the person sensitive to and aware of the negative impact of the particular behavior or attitude. This is usually done in an effort to help the person change and act in more positive ways or eliminate the particular behavior. Although you may be well intentioned, you probably will not realize that the self-absorbed person is indifferent and not at all concerned about the impact on other people unless that other person is perceived as being of higher status. They tend to dismiss whatever you say as a lack of your misunderstanding, that you are in error, or something similar. When confronted, the self-absorbed person is able to conceal or mask the true self, which is grandiose, is manipulative, is exploitive, and has an entitlement attitude and lacks the capacity for empathic understanding. All other people, who are considered by the self-absorbed person to be of lesser status can encounter the unrecognized masked true self frequently, sometimes on a daily basis. Perhaps the following example can illustrate:

You are in a relationship (love, work, or friendly) with someone whom you do not recognize as having considerable self-absorption. You may tend to ignore or dismiss any disquieting feelings you experience as the relationship unfolds and either blame yourself, or circumstances, or that person's past experiences for the upsetting behaviors and attitudes toward you. You make a lot of excuses and may try to be more empathic and conciliatory, but you continue to feel even more that the person dismisses, invalidates, and/or tries to minimize you. In an effort to preserve the relationship you decide to confront the person. However, when you do confront the person, it does not go well as whatever you say about them is turned back on you and you become even more angry, resentful, hurt, and the like. That person characterizes you as inadequate and as blaming others for your faults and mistakes, and makes other such demeaning comments. The confrontation that was supposed to be about the other person now has you as the focus and target, and this can end up with you feeling worse than you did before you started the confrontation.

This example for an ineffective confrontation is all too common and is almost guaranteed to happen when you try to confront a person with considerable self-absorption.

So far, the emphasis has been on why confrontation with a self-absorbed person is not likely to produce positive outcomes for you the confronter, nor will the other person change. An accompanying thought is what would be effective and produce a positive outcome. You may be better off if you do not confront, but to try and see the person as they are, to accept that what you are seeing is accurate about the person, to not expect or try to effect changes for the person, and to work on your need to have a relationship with this person. Realistic expectations for this relationship in the future are more of the same distressing behaviors and attitudes, and you may want to explore for yourself the benefits and costs for staying in the relationship. Just don't expect the other person to change as that is very unlikely.

Summary

Discussed in this chapter were the behaviors and attitudes that can signal self-absorption, and when many of these are present for an individual, these can be troubling for a relationship. It may be that the anxious person in your life have many or they have a few. What is important for you to understand and remember is that the person cannot see those aspects of their self just as you are unable to see them in yourself. Trying to make the other person aware of their self-absorbed behaviors is futile.

CHAPTER EIGHT

The Worrier and the Complainer

Previous chapters described the anxious person in general; suggested helpful responses to their concerns, both in the moment and for long term; identified how you can reduce negative impacts on yourself and not act caught up in their intense emotions; and discussed how their inner world contributes to their behavior and why they cannot see some aspects of themselves that can contribute to their anxiety. This chapter and the next chapter provide suggestions for how you can effectively respond to the anxious person in your life who could be described as a Worrier or a Complainer, and for the Micromanager and Nagger. The responses described differ depending on your role(s) and relationship with the anxious person who is a parent, a boss, a coworker, a friend, a spouse, or an intimate partner.

Relationships and Expectations

Essential to understanding and responding to the anxious person in your life is the quality of the current relationship you have with that person and your desire to continue and/or improve that relationship. My assumptions for all of the suggestions provided are that you value the current relationship, care for the person, and want to preserve the relationship and/or increase its quality. If these assumptions are not valid for you, and you do not value the relationship or care for the person, then the suggestions are not likely to be as helpful although some could be of use to maintain harmony.

All of the relationships where coping suggestions are presented differ in quality and kind. That is, your relationship with your parent will be different from that with your boss or coworker. As you read the suggestions, think about the extent to which you value the relationship with the anxious person in your life and want to maintain or even increase the quality of the relationship. If the relationship is important to you, to what extent do you want to maintain it, build it and/or make it stronger? Another way to phrase it is to ask yourself the questions, "What is this relationship doing to or for me?" and "How much energy and time do I want to give to the relationship?"

Another consideration will be your expectations of reciprocity; that is, do you have expectations that your time, energy, and caring will be returned in some way to you, or do you give your time, energy, and caring to the anxious person in your life knowing that they will not reciprocate? Being altruistic and giving without an expectation of reciprocity is admirable but is not what is meant. The task is to identify if you expect reciprocity from that person and if you receive it. If so, what feelings arise from that, or, if not, does that produce negative feelings about yourself or about the other person?

There is one last consideration presented, to reflect on the extent and/or limit of your responsibility for the anxious person's well-being and/or welfare. Is it reasonable to expect that you have responsibility for any or all of the following for your anxious person? Do you feel a responsibility to take actions to ensure that

They do not suffer discomfort and that you care for their physical, emotional, or psychological well-being

Their moods or other feeling states do not allow them to be depressed or down

You take care of their comfort even at the expense of yours

You are acting in accord with their wishes and demands even if these are unspoken or assumed to be known by you

Their problems are solved

That the decisions they make are "right" or "good"

They do not suffer consequences for their actions

Since this book is written for adults and about adults, your responsibilities and any limits are not intended for children or for adults who may be impaired or for whom you do have responsibility because they cannot adequately care for themselves. You may have extensive responsibilities in these cases and fewer limits to the extent of your responsibilities.

Some General Characteristics of Anxious People

All categories for anxious people have some characteristics in common, such as the following:

Insatiable—can never be satisfied

Constantly anxious—they have few periods where they are not worried, complaining, micromanaging, or having something to nag about

Tend to be needy and clingy and want extensive reassurance

Observe few personal limits on who they express their anxiety to or about, and/or tend to be intrusive

Seem to be indifferent to the impact of their anxiety on others

Cannot effectively use self-soothing techniques or do not use them

Appear to want others to know how much they are suffering and the unfairness of this

It can seem that the anxious person in your life is *insatiable* and can never get enough reassurance, encouragement, support, attention, admiration, understanding, or of having someone to listen to their rants, venting, kvetching, and the like. Even when they are effective, solve their own problems, or everything is going well, they seem to be able to find something unacceptable, fantasize about possible happenings, cannot have enough order, or feel a lack of control. Never enough is a guiding principle for them.

Their anxiety seems to be *constant* even if or when they appear to manage and contain it. They can live in a state of constant apprehension always fearing the worst will happen and that they will be criticized or blamed. They do not feel adequate to be effective regardless of all of the evidence that they are able to be effective and have been effective. It is probably the constant expressions of their anxiety that can get to you and produce irritation and exasperation. Their anxiety seems to be deep, wide, never ending, and always with them.

Anxious people are *not always circumspect* about sharing their worries and concerns. They can also be intrusive when their need to express their anxiety allows them to be indifferent to what other people may be experiencing at that time. They will interrupt others just to express their anxiety, and, sometimes, this expression can take considerable time. They can expect that their relationship with you means that you will drop whatever you are doing and listen to them, let them take as much of your time as they need or want, and are happy or pleased to do so.

Many anxious people seem to be *needy and clingy*, and in constant need of reassurance. They tend to get upset at the least little things such as setbacks that can be anticipated and are not major, changes in schedules, not being able to find what they were looking for at a store, and other such glitches. Whereas many or most people cannot let minor glitches bother them and adjust, your anxious person does not seem to be able to do this and, in addition, has to let you and others know what they are enduring, how they are suffering and should be admired for putting up with this, and/or that you should act promptly to take care of them. This is where you come in. They seem too often turn to you for reassurance, and you try to provide that, but many are also thinking that they should or can provide some or much of this for themselves.

As noted previously, some anxious people seem to be or are *indifferent to the impact* of their anxiousness on others. They do not appear to care that their constant need for venting, fussing, and having to have things just so and so on can be irritating or demeaning or even offensive to another person. They are so intent on getting their needs or desires met immediately that they do not concern themselves with what this may be doing to the other person and their feelings, time, and activity. They seem to feel free to interrupt and disrupt others without concern for what impact it has on the other person. While the anxious person in your life may not be so self-centered at other times, when they become anxious, they seem to be self-focused and indifferent to the impact they have on you.

Many people manage their anxiety better than the anxious person does in your life because they developed *self-soothing actions* to give them balance and allow them to be more centered and grounded. What do you do when you find yourself becoming anxious? Do you worry, start complaining, micromanaging, or nagging? If so, what makes you stop and take steps to soothe yourself and/or the situation? Assuming that what is happening is not a crisis where prompt action is needed, you use self-soothing techniques and strategies. However, the anxious person in your life either doesn't have these or does not see them, and, thus, they become anxious and try to relieve their anxiety by unloading on you and/or others.

Either consciously or unconsciously, the anxious person in your life makes sure that you and *others stay aware of their suffering*. For example, they can make comments and remarks to tell you the following:

How much they have to endure that is distressing for them.

The unfairness or selfishness of others that is causing them to have to be worried, complain, micromanage, or nag.

Comments such as "I always have to be the one who ensures that things are done right, stay on top of the task so that it gets done, and so on." Or asking, "Why do I have to be the one who does?"

I can't catch a break.

It's one problem after the other, and I'm the one who has to worry about (nag/complain/manage) it.

Everyone encounters problems and glitches but not everyone feels completed to have others know just how much they have to endure or suffer.

Presented were a couple of basic thoughts to keep in mind as you read the suggestions for coping with the anxious person in your life, the kind and quality of the relationship with your anxious person, and the expectations they may have for you and your responses. We now move to providing more specific suggestions for the Worrier and the Complainer.

The Worrier

Review the following characteristics to determine the extent to which the anxious person in your life is a Worrier. Rate each characteristic as 5—almost always; 4—very often exhibits this; 3—often exhibits this; 2—seldom exhibits this; 1—never or almost never exhibits this (Table 8.1).

Some Worriers can be very imaginative, and while there can be some reality about their worries, there can also be some fantasy as they can readily think of all kinds of things that could or even could not happen. Sometimes, there does not seem to be any outer limits for what they imagine and usually fear could happen. There may be times when they react to their imagined fears rather than more realistic fears.

Worriers tend to react easily to their experiencing, their imagination, or information from outside sources, and it can appear that sometimes they react to things that we don't begin to know or to understand. They can see implications and make inference about almost anything, which can make it difficult for you at times to follow their thought process to help you understand why they are reacting as they are.

Probably, what can puzzle you or try your patience is when they are worried but cannot pinpoint the worry, or when what they seem to be worried about has little or no substance. They are worried to the extent that they are talking to you about their worry but cannot identify what they are worried about or why this is worrying them.

It can appear that no matter how competent, capable, or adequate your worries are, they still need constant reassurance, especially from you. Deep

Table 8.1 Worrier Scale

Worrier scale imaginative (e.g., seems to react to speculations)	5	4	3	2	1
1. Reacts easily	5	4	3	2	1
2. Tends to see "the worst-case scenario"	5	4	3	2	1
3. Can worry without having a specific to worry about	5	4	3	2	1
4. Seems to need constant reassurance	5	4	3	2	1
5. Uses few self-soothing strategies	5	4	3	2	1
6. Gets easily frustrated	5	4	3	2	1
7. Talks a lot about trivial concerns	5	4	3	2	1
8. Is reluctant to rely on others to follow through	5	4	3	2	1
9. Seems to react to imagined terrors, negative possibilities, and the like	5	4	3	2	1
10. Stays on edge, anticipating problems	5	4	3	2	1

Scoring: Add your ratings to obtain a total score. The total score can indicate the intensity of the Worrier. Use the following as a guide:

46–55	A very intense Worrier
36–45	An intense Worrier
26–35	Somewhat intense Worrier
16–25	Worries but not intense
6–15	Little intensity

down, they may not believe in the validity of the evidence or fear that they cannot maintain what they have, for example, competence; that others will outdo or exceed or become better than they can do; or that they are unaware of or missing something important to their continued survival.

Self-soothing strategies are usually learned or developed early in life, but some people do not either learn or fail to use these. The Worrier in your life does not adequately use self-soothing strategies, logical self-talk, or a thought-stopping technique or other distractions to become calmer or more centered and grounded and thereby be more able to manage their worry. If you were to ask them how they manage their worry, it's very likely that they would note that talking (off-loading it) to you is the preferred way. Chapter 10 presents some self-soothing strategies you can model for your anxious person in the hope that they may try one or more.

Worriers seem to be easily frustrated. The slightest glitch can have them imagining all kinds of dire possibilities. Some adopt a "The sky is falling" attitude, which helps increase their anxiety. Glitches, barriers, or other constraints are irritating to many but not as frustrating as these are for the Worrier who can be more intensely affected by these. Any glitch produces a dire chain of events, real but usually imaginary, that leads to failure, blame, and/or criticism, and that is intolerable. In addition, there seems to be no end to the list of things, actions, or people that can produce frustration for the Worrier.

Things that can seem trivial to many people can loom large and important to the Worrier, and, thus, they can discuss, describe, and recount these trivial matters in great detail. It's not that these things don't have any value or interest as they may have some; it's more that they need to talk with you for extended periods of time regardless of interrupting or disrupting you. While there may be some deeper significance to their concern that seem trivial to you, ferreting out the deeper concern or association is probably not something you are trained or qualified to do and is not recommended as a strategy that is helpful for them or for the relationship.

Almost everyone values dependability and reliability as these reduce uncertainty and produces confidence that tasks and other commitments will be supported. All of us have likely encountered situations where others, people, institutions, or even the forecasts for weather are not reliable or dependable. We hope for these but are able to adjust many times when something or someone doesn't act so. The Worrier, on the other hand, has encountered lack of dependability and reliability enough so that they do not trust anyone or anything to be dependable or reliable. The disappointments they have experienced has produced a reluctance to trust that others can ever be reliable or dependable so that when they cannot control everything or everyone, this produces great anxiety for them.

The Worrier seems to stay on edge much or all of the time. Even if they seem to be relaxing, they can quickly switch to the intensely worried mode. They can be good at anticipating potential problems, and this is very helpful in preventing them. Some of their worries are based in reality on their past experiences and/or on information and knowledge that allows them to sometimes better anticipate constraints, barriers, and other problems. Just remember, however, that they can be under considerable stress trying to stay on top of potential problems, unanticipated glitches, and imagined negative possibilities.

Helpful Reactions and Strategies

An earlier chapter discussed some general responses for an immediate and current interaction, and another chapter provided some suggestions for the long term for the anxious person in your life. Following are some reactions and strategies geared toward the anxious person who can be described as a Worrier. Any of the suggestions are actions to avoid as these can be common responses that are not helpful. We'll begin with three actions to avoid.

Do not minimize or dismiss their imaginary or seemingly impossible concerns and possibilities.

Do not suggest solutions or fixes or give advice.

Do not follow or explore their speculations, for example, "what if"?

The Worrier, whether an intimate partner, coworker, boss, or friend, will not respond positively when you minimize or dismiss their concern no matter how far-fetched that may be. Yes, you may be correct in your evaluation and judgment about the perceived possibilities, but if you convey this to your Worrier, they are more likely to feel that you are minimizing or dismissing them. In other words, while you are focusing on the content, they are focusing on their selves and feeling as if you are discounting them as a person. You are focusing on cognitive concerns while they are focusing on emotional concerns.

Even when you think you have a solution or a "fix" for the concern, or have some advice for them, it is best that you do not offer that. When you give advice, it may be that the advised action will be acted on and not work out well, in which case you will be blamed. If the advice does work out to the Worrier's satisfaction, that is reinforcement for them to come to you even more often with their concerns, as you have demonstrated that you can solve the problem or "fix" what needs fixing in their eyes. It is also possible that your advice, when acted on and well intentional, can result in someone else's distress or discomfort because the Worrier in your life did not give you accurate and complete information. It may be best that you refrain from giving advice.

Since Worriers can be very imaginative and fanciful, they are apt to speculate a lot. Following their line of thought and exploring their speculations are time consuming and unproductive because much is unknown in any speculation about anything, and there is the risk of acting on the "what if?" that will produce negative outcomes. The Worrier in your life is likely able to produce numerous "what ifs?" for just about anything, and you have to decide if you want to join the speculations or try to direct time to be more realistic and logical. Joining with them to explore their speculations is encouragement for them to do this with you more frequently and maybe in greater detail. This can be a considerable time eroder.

Let's turn to describing some techniques that may be helpful to use in interactions with the Worrier in your life.

Stay calm and consciously focus on your breathing.

Stay mindful of the limits of your personal responsibilities.

Listen for the core concern and restate that.

Encourage and reaffirm your faith in their ability to find their own solutions.

Your calmness when confronted with the Worrier's concerns cannot be overly emphasized. Your calmness helps bring the interaction to the present, can assist to center and ground both of you, and conveys that things are under control or they will be controlled. To help becoming calm, you can consciously focus on your breathing and ensure that it is deep and even. You are also modeling how they can use a self-soothing technique that will help calm, center, and ground them.

It is also beneficial if you can remain mindful of the limits of your personal responsibility for the Worrier in your life as was discussed in Chapter 4. No matter how close or intimate the relationship is with your Worrier, there are still limits for the extent to which you are responsible for their well-being, moods, solving their problems for them, or ensuring that they do not become distressed or upset. An incomplete understanding of where you end and where they begin contributes to you becoming enmeshed or overwhelmed with their concerns and feelings. You may need to remind yourself on occasion especially if you get caught up in their emotional intensity. You can be of more help to the Worrier in your life when you recognize and act in accord with your personal limits for them.

Most helpful in interactions with almost everyone and especially for the Worrier in your life is when you can listen without judging, interrupting, or offering advice or your solutions. The suggestion here is that you listen to understand the core concern and that you reflect or restate it. Listening in this way means that you are not thinking about your response or other personal things, that you are focused on the speaker, that you separate out facts and other realistic parts of the message, that you don't get caught up in the speaker's emotional intensity, and that you identify fluff from substance. Listening in this way means that you:

Orient your body to the speaker and look at them; you can always turn or look away if needed

Focus on the speaker

Hear the words and unspoken feeling

Identify the central or main point as the speaker sees it

Accept that their emotional intensity may be interfering with their judgment and perceptions

The final step is to reflect the Worrier's core concern that is based on reality and on facts. For example, if the core concern as you understand it is that someone *might* or *could* do something that is not factual, it is speculation. If, however, the core concern is a fact such as their mother's operation is scheduled for the next morning and they are fearful of the results, those are factual and can form the reflective response. In the latter case, it is important that the reflective response not minimize the fear.

Encourage the anxious person to try and develop their own solutions to their concern and affirm your confidence in their ability to do so. In other words, do not quickly give them advice as to what they should do or think. Rather, try asking them what would be their desired outcome, and then ask what options or alternatives they have considered. Guiding them in this way encourages them to think instead of getting caught up in their intense feelings, can help decrease some of the emotional intensity, and is affirming of your confidence in their abilities. Do not rush to give your thoughts, ideas, reactions, or solutions. They are too focused on their experiencing to make much sense of what you are saying. All of these suggestions assume that there is not a crisis where immediate action is needed.

A Process for the Anxious Worrier

The two basics to keep in your thoughts when choosing a strategy for the anxious person in your life who is a Worrier are the closeness of the relationship and the kind of worry or concern being presented to you. Use the following scale in Table 8.2 to help in your decision about responding. Rate the relationship from 5—extremely important to

Table 8.2 Importance of Relationship and Worry Scale

Parent	1	2	3	4	5
Spouse/partner	1	2	3	4	5
Friend/family member	1	2	3	4	5
Boss/supervisor	1	2	3	4	5
Coworker	1	2	3	4	5

Now rate the importance of the worry being presented using the scale 5—realistic, possible, and critical; 4—possible but not critical; 3—unlikely but possible; 2—unlikely; 1—fantasized (exaggerated)

Parent	5	4	3	2	1
Spouse/partner	5	4	3	2	1
Friend/family	5	4	3	2	1
Boss/supervisor	5	4	3	2	1
Coworker	5	4	3	2	1

A rating of 5 indicates that you highly value the relationship and the worry is real and acute.

A rating of 4 indicates that you value the relationship and the worry, while possible, is not critical at this point.

A rating of 3 indicates that the relationship is a cordial one but not a close one and that the worry is somewhat unimportant at this time.

A rating of 2 or 1 for the relationship indicates that you have no emotional investment in the relationship and that the worry is not realistic nor important.

you; 4—very important to you; 3—important to you; 2—little importance to you; and 1—not important to you.

Let's assume that the relationship and the worry being presented are rated 3 or above and you want to preserve the relationship as is or even increase its value to you. The following sequence will be a positive strategy for you to use:

Use your emotional insulation

Breathe and remain calm

Listen even if you have to mentally set a time limit; reflect their feelings about the concern

Decide if the worry is short or long term

Solicit their thoughts about possible solutions

By the time you work through the sequence, their emotional intensity is reduced, you did not catch their feelings, you reaffirmed the importance and quality of the relationship for you, and they may have found their own solutions or recognized that their worry was not needed and/or not realistic.

The Complainer

The anxious person who carps, kvetches, and complains a lot and about almost everything is categorized here as the Complainer. Use the following rating scale in Table 8.3 to get a sense of the behaviors and attitudes that can characterize or describe them. Use the ratings of 5—always or almost always; 4—very often; 3—often; 2—seldom; 1—never or almost never

The attitude or belief that the Complainer has to ensure that things go "right" or "are right" is deeply ingrained for them and can be the basis for

Table 8.3 The Complainer Scale

1.	Seems to feel that they have to ensure that things are done "right."	5	4	3	2	1
2.	Think that their way is the best or only way to do or perceive things.	5	4	3	2	1
3.	Fusses, frets, and tends to talk a lot.	5	4	3	2	1
4.	Tends to personalize comments others make and/or their nonverbal behavior.	5	4	3	2	1
5.	Has little flexibility.	5	4	3	2	1
6.	Demonstrates little or no ability to manage transition.	5	4	3	2	1
7.	Looks for perfection.	5	4	3	2	1
8.	Tends to be overly reactive.	5	4	3	2	1
9.	Lacks judgment about the urgency, significance, and/or importance of situations or other things.	5	4	3	2	1
10.	Easily identifies flaws and imperfections.	5	4	3	2	1

Scoring: Add your ratings to get a total score.

46–55	A very intense Complainer
36–45	An intense Complainer
26–35	Somewhat intense Complainer
16–25	Complains but not always or intensely
6–15	Little complaining or intensity

much of their complaining. These people highly value and insist on order, predictability, and consistency and are convinced that they must ensure that everything meets those standards. Thus, they become very anxious when confronted with unpredictability, disorder, and inconsistency for fear of being blamed or criticized or even destroyed if others are displeased, inconvenienced, or inadequate. It's no wonder that they remain anxious because there is little that can be adequately predictable and put in order or where there are no inconsistencies, especially in our everyday lives where much of what we depend on is out of our control. However, the Complainer continues to act as if they did have control or could get control of just about everything.

A less endearing characteristic can be the Complainer's conviction and attitude that they know what is right or best for just about everyone and everything. They volunteer their advice and can become offended when others do not agree or have their own thoughts about what is right or best. In addition, some Complainers can complain about others who are not receptive to their advice or perceptions. Some can then complain that they are not listened to or respected for their superior wisdom and understanding.

A significant defining behavior of the Complainer is that they fuss a lot. Always fussing about something, they talk a lot. There may be times when others simply tune them out because the fussing is not about anything of significance, no response given seems to be satisfactory, and the listener feels in adequate to address the Complainer's concerns. If you are in a close relationship with the Complainer, they can interrupt their fussing to change you with not listening or caring about their concerns.

The Complainer can be very alert and sensitive to others' comments and nonverbal behaviors, tending to almost always personalize these as something negative about them. While they may be correct sometimes that these were personally directed toward them and were negative, they can also be wrong many times. It's not that they personalize these; they seem to also have the need to let you know what they object to in great detail. They dissect words, tone physical movements, and so on; speculate about the message and the other person's motives; and cannot consider that they may be overly reacting, misinterpreting what was said or done, or that it was negative or directed toward them. They continue to fuss, carp, and complain.

Rigid and inflexible are two descriptors for many Complainers. The least little glitch, unanticipated change, or any such need to be flexible seems to be very disconcerting for them. They cannot see other alternatives to what they had wanted, planned, or anticipated when that was not exactly what they faced. They cannot seem to accept alternatives and continue to insist on what they consider to be "right" or "best" *and* are not exactly reticent about making their thoughts known to others, usually you. You have probably realized that your suggestions for alternatives are not received well and tend to produce more complaints. The Complainer may think that they are voicing only their thoughts, but others see it as constantly complaining.

Transitions may be especially hard and stressful for the Complainer because they do not handle or manage these well. They become easily frustrated because transitions often mean ambiguity and uncertainty. There is not enough order, predictability, or consistency to comfort them. Thus, their complaints tend to increase in number and become more intense and frequent, and they find new things to complain about. Transitions mean change, and even positive changes seem to fuel their complaints.

In addition to valuing order and predictability, Complainers seem to be *seeking perfection* for everything and for everyone. They cannot or do not understand how others can tolerate or manage imperfection as they consider anything less than perfect as being shameful. Perfection is a worthy goal, and it can be enriching to oneself to achieve perfection in or for something as long as there is also an acknowledgment that perfection is an aspiration and is not always a necessity for one's positive self-esteem. It is also healthier and more rewarding to realize when something is acceptable or good enough. That does not mean that you stop trying to achieve perfection, just that it not be a constant expectation for you and everyone else, everything, or all of the time.

Many Complainers tend to be overly reactive. They are always alert for the least indication that something is not as it should or ought to be so that they can bring this to your and everyone's attention, or that they are being inconvenienced as not attended to as they would wish, or sometimes things, in general. They complain because they want you and everyone else to know just how much they are vigilant, observant, and upset, and that their world is not as it should be or wanted. Some Complainers expect you to take care of their complaints, and, if you cannot or don't do it to their satisfaction, that produces even more complaining. Depending on the relationship with the Complainer in your life, you may find that interactions about their complaints are more about their dissatisfaction with you and the relationship than it is about what they are complaining about.

Sometimes, it can seem that the Complainer magnifies the urgency and importance of their complaints. They can seem to complain about trivial things in a manner that suggests that it is of utmost importance to take care of this, whatever this may be, promptly. They can seem to be unable to distinguish between something that is both urgent and important, those things that are important but not urgent, those that are urgent but not important, and those that are neither important nor urgent and gauge what if any action is needed. Everything to them is both urgent and important and needs to be brought to your attention.

Some Complainers have an uncanny ability to see flaws and imperfections. This ability can be an asset for those engaged in quality control activities. However, for the majority of people, it is not helpful to have flaws and imperfections brought to their attention most or all of the time and about almost everything. The Complainer may have an erroneous belief that others want to know about everything that they consider to be flaws and imperfections so that these can be fixed, even those about which nothing can be done. Even telling them that they don't need to report on every flaw or imperfection, or that you cannot fix everything, does not deter them from continued complaints.

A Process for the Anxious Complainer

Probably the most important points are that the Complainer is unlikely to change and not complain so much. Just accept that they are wired to want and expect order, predictability, and consistency and that their complaints are their way of trying to get this or these. Given that they will continue to complain, what follows are some suggestions for you to lessen the impact of their incessant complaints on you. Let's start with some actions to avoid as these are likely to produce even more complaints and/or negatively affect the relationship.

Actions to avoid:

Acting to "fix" the complaint almost always

Let their anxiety confuse you

Play one-upmanship

Suggest that the complaint is relatively minor

Provide advice or your solutions

Ignore, minimize, or downplay the complaint

Don't say "Look on the bright at side"

Do not ask "Why does this bother you?"

Unless it is your responsibility to "fix" the complaint, do not act on the complaint. When you act without having the responsibility, you reinforce the Complainer's tendency to point out what they object to because when they do, you act to fix it or make it better. Your tendency to get on their complaints then becomes their expectation and can cause the complaining to increase.

It is important that you do not let their anxiety confuse you and you can get confused because they can give you nonessential information along with the complaint. It is much more helpful for you to focus on the essential matter and tune out the clutter noise and irrelevant details. It is also helpful to verbalize the central and important information.

Don't play one-upmanship. It can be tempting to point that doing so can irritate and frustrate them. They can then also start playing that game, and then both of you become frustrated at trying to decide who has it worse.

Do not say anything that indicates that their complaint is relatively minor or that other people in the world are worse off than they are. You may be correct as this is usually true, but that sentiment is like throwing gasoline on a fire. What that maybe realistic appraisal does is to convey that they and their complaint are unimportant to you, that they are being whiney, and that you are not interested in their well-being. Notice that the outcomes are all about them and your relationship with them. So, if you value the relationship, don't say this.

Try to refrain from providing your solutions. Yes, you may know what they can do to address their complaints, but your solutions may not fit them for one reason or another. The Complainer does not want you to only solve this particular complaint; they want you to ensure order, predictability, and consistency for everything and always. This is why they keep looking to you to solve their complaints. If you are in the habit of trying to provide solutions for the Complainer in your life, you may want to consider reducing or eliminating your need and/or attempts to give these.

It can be tempting at time to ignore, dismiss, or minimize their complaints, but doing so is not helpful to the relationship. Even if the relationship is not close or valued, you may be in a position where you need to preserve the relationship such as with a coworker or have other reasons to maintain harmony and cordiality. There are more positive actions you can take that will both preserve the relationship and allow you to better cope with their anxiety.

You may have the best intentions but try to not say anything that suggests that they look on the bright side, or that there is something positive about the complaint. That may be our tendency or approach to glitches and the like, but the Complainer is not like you in this respect. They are more likely to do the opposite and become offended because you are not taking them seriously enough in their eyes. The old saying that misery loves company is more applicable than finding a silver lining. Do not ask the Complainer why something bothers them. Why questions are not helpful and doing so this can suggest to them that you don't agree, you don't see what is wrong, and they are wrong for complaining; none of this will be helpful for the relationship or the interaction. You are more likely to intensify their irritation.

There are also six more constructive actions you can take: assess, sympathize, lament, encourage, support, and/or distract. Assess the validity of the complaint; its importance, both for now and for the future; the extent of the personal discomfort it is presenting; and the need for action. Many of the Complainer's complaints may be valid, but not all of them as they can be as prone to misunderstanding and misperceptions as are other people. Some complaints are not valid. In addition, assess the importance of the complaint, even valid ones. The problem can be valid but still not be very important. Note the extent or degree to which the problem is causing distress either to the Complainer or to others as this helps you determine what if any action needs to be taken. You now can have enough information to judge if you need to act, in which case you will then act to resolve the complaint.

If, as may be the case most often, you do not need to take action, your next step is to sympathize. That is, you join with the Complainer in the "Gee, isn't that awful," and lament that they are having to put up with or endure whatever the complaint is about. Agree that it is not right, that it is happening, and that they are affected. However, do not take action to try and resolve or fix it. The joining by sympathizing and lamenting reaffirms the relationship and that you do care about them. Encourage the Complainer to find their solution. Ask what they want to do about it and keep the focus on them acting. The solution should not call for you or someone else to act. If the action to resolve or correct the complaint is the responsibility of someone else, their action can be to bring it to that person's attention, but not for you to do that. In one way, you are encouraging the Complainer to become more resourceful and less dependent on you and others to take care of them.

Support their decision about their action whether that is to do nothing or to act. You may not agree with what they propose to do but don't discourage that decision unless what they propose to do would be harmful or detrimental. In which case, you can try to use the next strategy, distracting them. However, even if you see a better way or a better solution, try to encourage your Complainer to find their own solutions and support their decision.

The final strategy is to distract the Complainer. Don't overuse their strategy because if it is used too often, it will become infective. Examples for distractions are as follows:

Call attention to something unusual in the immediate environment.

Interject and note there is something you forgot or meant to tell them.

Ask for information or their opinion about something you feel certain that they know.

Suggest that you need an urgent bathroom break and go.

Propose something pleasurable such as a walk, getting a beverage, or doing something easily available.

The six strategies can be used with the Complainer no matter the closeness of the relationship. The important points to remember are to not tune them out, hear the complaint but don't feel compelled to take action, and reaffirm your confidence in their capability to take care of their complaints. While the Complainer may never fully stop complaining, your understanding can help reduce the number and intensity of their complaints.

CHAPTER NINE

The Micromanager and the Nagger

Another two categories for an anxious person are the Micromanager and the Nagger. Both are expecting other people to do what they want to be done, to do it promptly, and, in the case of the Micromanager, to do it a certain way. Both are anxious that they be perceived as more than adequate and admired. They are almost always concerned about themselves even when they may think or rationalize what they are demanding of others is what is needed, is best for the other, and is "right." Their anxiety stems from fears of being perceived as shameful and inadequate and they strive for perfection from others so that they can be perceived favorably.

Indeed, they can be often perceived favorably as their efforts at micromanaging and/or nagging tend to pay off as others do respond as they desire them to, and they do tend to get the job or task accomplished. The residual feelings left with other people they live or work or interact with may not be so positive. Let's take a look at some of their behaviors and attitudes, and then at suggestions for coping with these and for managing your reactions. We will first describe the Micromanager and provide some suggestions and then address the Nagger.

The Micromanager

The Micromanager tends to every aspect and detail for a job or task with extensive descriptions of what they think needs doing and why, followed by frequent checks on you, in-depth questioning of how and why you did or did not do something, can be thrown off-guard or disconcerted by others' ideas or any disruptions to their plans for you to carry out, and seems to expect prompt and complete compliance with their orders or desires. They will interrupt your wok with their demands for an immediate and complete update on your progress, some will intervene and take over the work while insisting that you watch them so that you can do it the "right" way, and also have the expectation that you will be appreciative of what they are doing for you, all of which can be irritating and demoralizing.

Following are some behaviors that the Micromanager may display. Rate the Micromanager in your life using the rating: 5—extremely like the person; 4—very much like the person; 3—frequently like this; 2—seldom like this; 1—never or almost never like this.

Table 9.1 The Micromanager Scale

1.   Considers almost all mistakes as preventable.

2.   Thinks that others cannot be trusted to do it "right."

3.   Feels that others are not reliable or dependable.

4.   Knows how whatever it is should or ought to be done.

5.   Tends to be nit-picking.

6.   Frequently checks on your progress.

7.   Wants things done "their way."

8.   May not be organized.

9.   Checks and rechecks to ensure that you are correct or that what you are doing is "right."

10. Can hover over you and watch intently while you work.

11. Mistrusts any communication that is not face to face.

12. Has a strong emotional investment in the outcomes of the task or job.

Scoring: Add your ratings to derive a total score. Use the total score to determine the extent to which the person is a Micromanager.

48–60	Very much Micromanages
36–47	Often Micromanagers
24–35	Tends to Micromanage but not as often
12–23	Seldom Micromanages
0–11	Never, or almost never Micromanages

Descriptions for the Micromanager

All Mistakes Are Preventable

No one likes mistakes or sets out to make mistakes, but these do happen, and many can be fixed. A Micromanager can assume that all mistakes are preventable and that their diligent attention can prevent these even when those that are other people's responsibilities and to not prevent mistakes is shameful. They can feel ashamed for their and others' mistakes and work hard to prevent them.

Now, you may think or react to the Micromanager as if they are trying to tell you how to do something you know how to do, or one where you would like to figure it out for yourself, but they are interrupting, and you see their efforts as undermining you. This is one reason that you can become irritated at that person. You can wish that the person would first leave you alone, let you work or do what is necessary, and ask for help when you think you need it. The Micromanager may even say to you that they are trying to prevent mistakes.

Suggestion: Agree that you also want to prevent mistakes, appreciate their efforts at prevention, and ask for help when a mistake is possible. Do not say you will ask them for help when needed.

Trusting Others

The Micromanager is anxious because they do not trust others to do what is needed without constant attention and direction. Although their previous experiences may have led them to this perception where others failed to do what was needed or expected, they may also have this mindset regardless of previous experiences. Or, your Micromanager may have both the mindset and their experience.

The important thing for you, however, is to remember that the Micromanager cannot or does not trust others to do what is needed without managing them, and this perception is not personal because of you. No matter how good at the task or job you are or have been shown to be, they cannot let go of their need to micromanage and, even in some cases, to recognize others' capabilities and competencies. Even if you were to verbalize their lack of trust for you noting of evidence to the contrary, they will deny this or be unable to see it or think that you are attacking them without reason.

Suggestion: Never confront them with their mistrust of you, or lack of confidence in your capabilities as this would not be likely to be received or responded to very well. You may just have to accept that they are mistrustful and not take it as being personal.

Reliability and Dependability

I'm sure that you appreciate people who are reliable and dependable as these are the people who follow through on their responsibilities, obligations, and promises. You are fortunate if you have several of these people in your life. The Micromanager may also have people in their lives who are reliable and dependable, appreciate them, but can still be anxious that they will not be consistently reliable or dependable. The Micromanager is alert to any hint or fantasized hint that you may not be totally reliable or dependable in all circumstances and situations. They cannot understand that there may be events or other unanticipated actions that could or did impact you so that you could not follow through for that one time. The Micromanager then expands even one lapse as being the default and then assumes that you are never to be relied on or depended on unless they keep tabs on you.

Suggestion: Keep them informed about your progress before they check on you.

Should and Ought

The Micromanager knows how things should or ought to be done—it doesn't matter what it is or what your capabilities are—and they are quick to share this information with you, sometimes in detail and in specific context. The good part is that they can know and understand the task in detail, but the other part is that they want you to follow their instructions and tend to present these as dictates; that is, you should or ought to do what they tell you to. Many times, they will use those words, should and ought, ignoring the possible negative reactions others can have when told what they should or ought to do. Sometimes other people want to do it their way, can feel that the Micromanager is putting them down or have a perception that they are stupid, or hear a parent's voice that arouses negative memories and feelings. Few people react positively to being told what they should or ought to do. They may tend to use "should" and "ought" in other parts of their lives and do not understand why they get the negative reactions that they do.

Suggestion: Try to not overreact to their use of should and ought, or to try to get them to give you more leeway to do it as you want to. Depending on the relationship, you could ignore their dictate and do it your way, or better, do it their way so that they will not have any comeback if their way does not work or work as well.

"Nitpicks"

Nitpicks is a term generally used to describe someone who is fussy about the tiniest detail about almost everything. They may also "pick" at things that are irrelevant and unimportant to the point where you just want to say, "Enough already." This tendency may come from an excessive focus on details, an inability to distinguish what is important and what is not, and the drive for perfection. The Micromanager cannot accept that something good enough can be acceptable at times and continues to prod others to get to their perception of perfection. While some attention to details can be rewarding, his excessive and continual picking at the tiniest detail, which mostly is irrelevant and unimportant, can be very irritating.

Suggestion: Ignore this as much as possible or agree that they are correct and try not to get frustrated.

Check on Progress

The Micromanager can become very anxious when they are away from the task as they do not know what you are doing. Don't forget that they only trust themselves to be reliable, to be dependable, and to do it right. Hence, they have this need to check on you over and over again. They cannot rest at all until they know exactly what is going on with you or the task. This need to know exactly leads them to engage in frequent check-ins, extensive questioning of you, and even telling you how to do something that you know very well how to do. They are trying to take care of their anxiety by checking and rechecking on you. You may find that trying to avoid the frequent checks does not work as they can be driven to make sure that things are going as they want them to go and will continue to search for you to do the check-in. In addition, they will then fuss or chide you for not being available when they wanted to check in with you.

Suggestion: If possible, give a daily report on your progress.

"Their Way"

The Micromanager has a conviction that their way of thinking, perceiving, and acting is exemplary and that other should recognize this and do things their way. In some ways, the Micromanager can consider others as extensions of their selves and thereby as under their control so that others should be doing things the Micromanager's way. Some Micromanagers may be in a position of authority where they can say and enforce, "My way or the highway." Certainly, many micromanaging parents and bosses, and some spouses or intimate partners, are in this position. While there can be some positives to doing things the Micromanager's way, they often ignore or overlook the negative fallout from this perspective and conviction.

There are situations where this perspective and conviction can be helpful, and I don't want to overlook mentioning some of these:

Surgeons who are in the process of operating

Coaches during a game

Directors of performances, for example, music and drama

Supervisors who are trying to prevent physical accidents

Emergency responders to life-threatening situations

The military in combat

If you notice, all the examples involve immediate responses where it is essential or helpful to do what the in-charge person or lead tells you to do or expects you to do in order to accomplish the task and ensure a positive outcome.

Suggestion: Unless it bothers you, try to do most things "their way." If "their way" isn't the most effective, efficient, or workable, that will be evident.

Not Organized

It seems to be an oxymoron that the Micromanager can be ordered and detail oriented and, at the same time, not be organized. Think of it as their being focused on one thing in the midst of many things. That one thing consumes their attention, interest, and efforts, but they then lose sight of the big picture, which can result in their attention to details and order as they see them but not being organized otherwise. For example, the Micromanager may know what needs to be done but do not ensure that all needed materials are available at different times when they are needed, or submit paperwork to get what is needed in a timely manner, or notify relevant personnel not directly involved when their input or expertise will be needed as when or how, and other such organizational matters. Another example is when the Micromanager tends to be neat but unorganized. Yes, their desks or other furniture has neat piles or even no piles, but they are unable to find materials when wanted or needed because the piles are not organized in any particular order or way. These piles are neatly aligned, not scattered, which gives an illusion of being organized, but when something needs to be found that cannot be easily or promptly done. Of course, if the Micromanager has a helper, that person can keep them organized.

Suggestion: Ignore as much as possible.

Checking and Rechecking

The continuous internal anxiety of the Micromanager compels them to check on you or on other details and to recheck at frequent intervals. This person is also trying to be helpful or, at least that is how they rationalize their actions. On some level, they realize what they are doing but do not seem to be able to prevent themselves from checking and rechecking. They want to ensure that you are doing what is needed, doing it as specified by them, to take care of glitches as they cannot be sure that you can be counted on to know what to do if there is a glitch, but most of all to reassure themselves and quiet their internal anxiety.

What can be frustrating for you are the interruptions, disruptions, repetition of their directions, and the need to attend to their unnecessary anxiety. You want whatever it is to be done, done well, and correctly, but the constant checks are making it difficult for you to maintain your focus as is needed because you have to stop and try to calm or satisfy their anxiety for the moment as you will now that they will return over and over again.

Suggestion: Find a place to work where you are less likely to be disturbed or interrupted. If this is not possible, then breathe deeply and try to tolerate the interruptions as best as you can.

Hovering

In addition to checking and rechecking, the Micromanager tends to hover over you. Sometimes they will intently watch you as you are working, particularly if the work involves tools, manipulations of any kind, and even when you are working on the computer, which can be disconcerting and unnerving. If challenged about their hovering, they usually assert that they can quickly intervene if needed, or they can help you do whatever you are doing better or more efficiently, or that they just want to help. They may really believe that they are being helpful even when someone tells them that their hovering is not helpful, or that you will ask for help if needed. Their anxiety helps them deny that they are being unhelpful, disruptive, annoying, or pushy. Even when they try to resist hovering, they tend to return to doing so as that helps calm some of their anxiety.

Suggestion: Stand up to listen to them. They can't hover if you are standing as well as they can when you are sitting. Don't have anything in your hands, and just stand there. You cannot work when you have to stand and listen to the Micromanager, and they will quickly realize this.

Face-to-Face Communications

The Micromanager usually does not trust communications that are not in person and face-to-face. They mistrust written, phone, two-way radio, e-mail, text, or other forms of communications. They have a perception that only when they are present can communications be accurate. This mistrust may be based on experience but can also have a personal trait component where they are naturally suspicious and mistrustful. When experience is combined with a natural trait of suspicion and mistrust, it becomes easier to understand why they are anxious when communications are not face-to-face and even to better understand why they have this strong need to micromanage.

Suggestion: Try to limit the number of face-to-face communications you have with them each day, but also try to make a point of having at least one of these.

Emotional Investment

Must of the material presented to this point supports the idea that the Micromanager has an emotional investment in the job or task. It's almost as if the job or task is an integral part of the person and thereby is valued and cherished. When you can accept the extent and level to which the Micromanager in your life is emotionally invested in tasks and/or jobs, you will find that you are better able to tolerate their intrusive behaviors. You realize that their need to interfere is more about them than it is about anyone else or the task/jobs.

Some Micromanagers can fear that they are frequently being judged negatively by others, and micromanaging is their way of ensuring that others judge them favorably. Their reaction to this fear is to meddle in every aspect of what is being done so as to ensure that others have a positive opinion of them. Since every task/job has a significant emotional investment for them and they fear that they will be negatively judged, they are very attentive to even the smallest detail that may be irrelevant or that others could easily manage.

Another indicator of the Micromanager's emotional investment is the level of intensity they display when they "nitpick," or check and recheck about the same thing, their hovering, and so on. They are unable to relax or attend to other tasks or jobs until this one is completed to their satisfaction. They do not seem to be able to relax, to respond to humor, to notice or attend to others' concerns, to appear to value others' efforts or input, or to have the flexibility needed when things do not go exactly as they planned.

Suggestion: Try to be sensitive to how their emotional investment influences their interactions with you and with others, and keep the communication task focused, with progress reports.

Seven Strategies for Managing the Micromanager

In addition to the general strategies provided for all anxious people, there are seven strategies that may be helpful for the Micromanager in your life: updates, instructions, estimated completion, avoidance, remote communication, ask for what you need, and show appreciation. Judicious use of these strategies can help you while providing reassurance to them, which can help the Micromanager lower their anxiety and become calmer.

Provide Updates

Take the lead and provide frequent updates on progress and future plans for the task or job. In other words, don't wait for the Micromanager to interrupt you to ask for progress; give them a progress report before they have a chance to disrupt what you are doing as thinking. However, try to do this via phone, e-mail, or text, not in person. In fact, you may be able to propose to the Micromanager in your life that you can give updates and see if this will be sufficient to prevent them from checking and rechecking on you, or hovering. The downside can be that they don't get your updates frequently enough for their anxiety. The update could trigger their thought about additional work that needs to be done or if they are the kind of person who has to see for themselves will want to make a visit to you to see what you are doing. The kind and extent of the relationship you have with the person determines if frequent remotely communicated updates are sufficient enough to reduce some of the micromanaging or not.

Write Instructions

Since the Micromanager in your life is picky about details, is mistrustful of others' reliability and dependability, and has an emotional investment in the task or job and its outcomes, you may want to get in the habit of writing their instructions for what to do and how to do it no matter how trivial the task or how competent you are. Why go to this extent? Writing the instructions ensures a record of what you were told to do and how, provides an opportunity to clarify what they mean, and is a record if they should challenge you for not doing what you were supposed to do or not doing it "right."

You can also ask for instructions in writing or write them after a meeting with a copy of the Micromanager. These will be confirmation of what both of you understand to be the task and your responsibilities. You may think that you accurately remember and understand and, indeed, you may, but that doesn't mean that you and the Micromanager are on the same page or that your memories are as accurate as you wish. Instructions in writing can prevent misunderstands, inaccuracies, and maybe even some irritations.

Estimated Due/Completion Dates/Time

Whatever your responsibilities for task or job completion, make sure that you tell the Micromanager when you expect to complete your assignment or any part of it. Giving an estimated due/completion date/time may help forestall their need to hover or to keep checking especially if you are accurate in your time estimated. Another way is to ask them when they want it completed or partially completed or when they need an update on progress. And it is important that you try to meet these time estimates.

Disappear

There may be times when it is best for your mental health and for the relationship that you avoid the Micromanager, just for a little while but not for a long period of time. Yes, your disappearance can increase their anxiety, but you may need a short time-out in order to more effectively cope with them and their anxiety when you do reconnect. This is a time period where you can breathe and calm yourself, remind yourself of how you value the relationship, think of some of the suggested ways you can cope that are presented in this book, sequester yourself to finish what needs to be worked on, and other positive actions. You could take a walk, find a needed resource, talk or consult with someone, or even take a needed bathroom break.

Remote Communications

You can reduce your emotional catching when you use remote ways to communicate rather than face-to-face. Examples of remote communication include:

Telephoning including leaving a message

E-mail, especially if you keep it short and make it informative

Texting is helpful just to keep touch or to send short updates

Messaging on the computer or tablet a written note

Using these remote means of communication can provide some needed time-out while maintaining the connections and may be less anxiety producing for the Micromanager than the previously suggested tactic of disappearing.

Time and Space

An option is to ask for the time and space you need or want. Use this option carefully and with tact as the Micromanager may be likely to perceive your request as criticism of them. A message they can receive is that you don't want their assistance, which can produce hurt feelings on their part. How the request is received depends on their mood and level of anxiety, the relationship for the two of you, as well as how you phrase the request. Your level of frustration will also play a part in how you convey the message and how it may be received. While the task or job may be the priority for the Micromanager, the same may not be true for you and it may be helpful to remember that they are probably not aware of or sensitive to your needs or priorities. They can be very self-absorbed at times especially when their anxiety is intense.

Appreciation

Showing your genuine appreciation for their efforts to be helpful even when these are annoying and disruptive can contribute positively to the relationship. You know what that they think their intent is to be helpful, even if the intent produces irritation or frustration for you. This is an example for "They mean well," and at times, they are helpful. The essence of this suggestion is to be genuinely appreciative. You could do one of the following:

Smile at them and say, "Thanks"

Tell them that they are being helpful

Remark positively on their attention to detail

Say that you appreciate their attention

Complement them on their knowledge, directions, and so on

Showing some genuine appreciation at times can enrich the relationship. However, too much and/or too often can reinforce the micromanaging behavior, and you do want to prevent that. Strike a balance and be somewhat appreciative.

Micromanaging Your Life

Does the Micromanager in your life also try to micromanage your life by doing any of the following or something similar?

Telling you what clothes to wear

Telling you what clothes not to wear

Suggesting whom to be friendly with and whom to not be friendly with or shun

Frequently correcting your pronunciation and/or word choice

Straightening your apparel before you leave

Making negative comments about your appearance such as hair style

Telling you the "right" side of an argument or opinion or what to appreciate

Monitoring your behavior in social or other similar situations

Constantly telling you what you "ought" to think, feel, or do

Checking and rechecking to see if you followed their suggestions (dictates, orders, etc.)

It can seem at times that you are not able to meet their exacting standards or that they have a vision of what you are supposed to be and do that is inconsistent with whom you are, or that they are trying to make you over into their image. None of these possibilities are comfortable or helpful for the relationship and can cause a lot of friction. It can get to be a challenge at times to maintain or get your separateness and individuality.

You may find it helpful to understand their chaotic inner world; their intense need for orderliness, prediction, and control; and that their actions toward you are how they try to manage their anxieties. Knowing and understanding helps you to maintain your individuality and separateness as a unique individual, and to not get caught up in their anxiety and distress. In addition, you understand that you don't have to change to meet their demands as these are unlikely to be satisfied or cease. You will be better able to manage your feelings, set appropriate and firm boundaries that preserve both of you as separate and distinct, prevent you from catching their feelings and/or incorporating and acting on them, and you can develop effective responses to meet the various challenges they present. Using some of the suggested strategies and techniques may also be helpful.

The Nagger

One important thing to remember about the Nagger is that they never ever see themselves as nagging. Another point is that they become very offended at being termed a nag. These are important because what and how you communicate your perception of their actions and impact on you is critical for the relationship. While the Worrier, Complainer, and Micromanager tend to be aware of what they are doing and feeling, the Nagger tends to either be unaware or is too self-absorbed to realize how their actions are affecting you. Let's see if you have a Nagger in your life. Rate this person on each of the following behaviors and attitudes using the scale: 5—always or almost always; 4—very often; 3—often; 2—seldom; 1—never or almost never.

Table 9.2 The Nagger Scale

1.	Perceives themselves as helpful even when you ask them to stop reminding you of something.
2.	Does not want you or others to make mistakes or suffer consequences for those is their rationale for the frequent reminders.
3.	Chastises you and others when you don't do what they tell you to do.
4.	Has a tendency to know what is right, wrong for you, or what you should or ought to do.
5.	Tends to be concrete in giving orders, telling you what to do and the like.
6.	Perceives others as procrastinators, being trifling and lacking self-discipline.
7.	Fears that what you do or don't do is a negative reflection on them.

Scoring: Add your ratings to derive a total score. Use the total score to determine the extent to which the person is a Nagger

31–35	Tends to be a Nagger, and very often nags you
26–30	Often nags you and others
21–25	Will nag you and others at times
16–20	Seldom nags you or others
0–15	Never or almost never nags you or others

Try to Be Helpful

The Nagger is likely to have the mind-set that their constant reminders are helpful to others. They tend to be oblivious to the impact they are having on others or will dismiss others' protests. Your or others' negative reactions as not important as them as whatever it is that they want done is much more significant and important. It does not matter how small or unimportant what they want done may be, to them all tasks are urgent, important, and significant; thus, it is imperative that the task be accomplished for their benefit. They remain convinced that their constant reminders are helpful even if the receiver doesn't want them, may not need them, and certainly doesn't appreciate them, but they are convinced that what they are nagging about is essential for your well-being.

A gentle reminder can be helpful at times especially when you have a lot to do, or are otherwise engaged or distracted. That's when a reminder is appreciated. However, many Naggers don't seem to be able to restrict themselves to just one reminder, they have to say the same thing many times. Worse can be when you still forget and they can say that they told you to not forget. Generally, this is said with an air of superiority or exasperation, which conveys the implication that you are inferior and would be better off if you would listen to them and do what they tell you to do.

Prevent Mistakes or Consequences

This characteristic is usually perceived as a positive one where as it is helpful to prevent mistakes or suffering negative consequences. In Naggers' minds, they are helping to ensure that things go "right," and everything works well. Prevention of mistakes, lapses, and negative consequences can work well, so it is not so much that they are focused on prevention; it is the means they use in pursuit of it that tends to be the irritation.

It also doesn't help you to know that they are correct in what they are nagging about, and that you may drop the ball if you don't do what they are nagging you to do, or suffer unpleasant consequences. For example, you could be nagged to make an appointment with a doctor to have a mole checked. Delaying this could allow melanoma to grow more and making an appointment and keeping it could relieve your mind to find that it is benign. However, the nagging could be about something inconsequential where you can decide its importance to you and you don't need the Nagger's constant reminders. In addition, you may want to reflect on your need to be defiant when doing so is not in your best interest.

Chastise

The Nagger also tends to chastise you along with the reminders about the task. For example, a parent nagging their teen about hanging up a garment will also add words that are chastising, blaming, or critical of the teen such as, "Don't you ever consider that I have other things to do rather than having to pick up after you?" For some Naggers there is always a subtext message that the other person is inadequate, guilty of an offense, or is shameful. For some others, there is no subtext as they say this directly and then wonder why the relationship is negatively affected. This Nagger never seems to catch on what they are doing or saying is corrosive to the relationship and to the other person's well-being, no matter how correct the Nagger may be about the need for the task to be accomplished.

What can be infuriating is that the Nagger is chastising you just as a parent did when you were a child. You are now an adult and don't need or want to be treated like a child. Also, you don't want someone assuming a role like a parent and acting as if they have a right and responsibility to take charge of your actions, and to try and shame you into doing what they want you to do.

Right, Wrong, Should, Ought

Many who nag can have a mental vision or perception that they know:

What is "right" to do, to be, or to say for others

What is "wrong" and must not be said or done

What others "should" know, do, be, and say

How others "ought" to know better than to do, or say or even be

This internal vision fuels the nagging so that others' actions fulfill their inner need for order, predictability, and control. You may notice that the Nagger in your life seems to always have a real or valid explanation for why you and others are expected to act on their demands, and their explanation is usually some variation of doing what they think is right or wrong, or is something that you should, or ought to do.

The Nagger may tend to overlook, dismiss, or ignore the impact of their words and actions on others, can even be oblivious to how their words or actions are being received by others, or, in the case of some Naggers, do not care about the impact. They are more focused on getting you to do what they want or think that you "should" do to be concerned about your or anyone's reactions or feelings. Their constant nagging can be very corrosive to the relationship, but they are unlikely to notice or acknowledge that some are so convinced of their "rightness" that they do not see any validity in the receiver's reactions that are less than positive. They are "right" and you (and others) are "wrong."

There are very few of us who cannot use or appreciate reminders. However, the Nagger not only reminds you of things, but they can also be dedicated to minding your business whether you want them to or not. Their reminders are not just a one-time remark such as "Don't forget to"; they tend to repeat this over and over for one thing and for everything. It's almost as if they are trying to convince you of their importance in your life and for your well-being. You may be a well-functioning independent adult, but the Nagger in your life wants you to feel that they are indispensable and that you would not function very well without their reminders. This also fits with some Naggers minding your business where they want to know what you are doing, thinking, considering doing, and even your speculations so that they can tell you what you should or ought to do, and follow that up with constant nagging. So not only are they nagging you to do what they need to keep their world orderly, predictable, and under control, but they are also nagging you to do what they think you should do or be about things in your life that you can and do take care of by yourself.

Tend to Be Concrete

Concrete in this description refers to being specific, precise, and detailed. The Nagger can be impatient and unaccepting of anything that does not meet their internal exacting, but usually not specified standards and vision of what is "right" or "wrong" or "good" or "bad," and the like. They are usually not able to be accepting of anything that is good enough, for even small or unimportant or trivial things. They also notice small and irrelevant details and can insist that you and others take care of these to meet their exacting standards and, in addition will provide constant reminders. The Nagger also expects others to be as concrete and can become very upset at what they consider to be vague, ambiguous, or uncertain, which can lead to a whole new topic for nagging; that is, you and others must give them the precision, detail, and/or specificity they want and demand. They are very uncomfortable and cannot act at times when you or others are not as concrete as they wish or demand.

It is possible that the Nagger in your life does not understand or appreciate other personality traits such as being abstract or imaginative. They may not be able to fathom why everyone is not like them in being concrete and detail oriented. It could be that the Nagger doesn't recognize or accept how you may differ from them and may overlook what they consider to be obvious, or can ignore irrelevancies, and that you have a sense of what is most important and attend to this. This kind of difference and other differences that they do not understand could be a part of why they tend to nag you.

Perceptions of Others

The Nagger may not be aware of or admit that they tend to perceive others as procrastinators, trifling, and lacking self-discipline. This perception can then lead to their need and conviction that others need constant reminders for everything or almost everything. It's as if the Nagger feels superior because they meet their own exacting standards and others do not or cannot, which lead to their conclusion that others lack discipline. They are quick to pick up on others' procrastination, resistance, defiance, or just plain laziness about doing what the Nagger wants or demands that they do. Since the Nagger doesn't tend to forget and is relentless, those strategies do not halt nagging; they tend to increase it. In one sense, the Nagger has to have this negative perception of others in order to shore up their positive self-perception that they know what's right, wrong, good, or bad. They also seem to lack an appreciation for how you and others are distinct and separate individuals from them who may have other or more important priorities than taking care of their needs and demands.

Some Naggers seem to think that others should be more like they are, and if others are not like them in ways that they think are important, then others need to change to be more like the Nagger. They can have a mind-set that others need more self-discipline and that their nagging is their way to show them what they need to do to be more self-disciplined. These Naggers seem to ignore that others can differ from them in important ways and are also worthwhile as separate and distinct individuals, and their understanding of self-discipline may be flawed. None of this helps the relationship with you.

Your Actions or Inactions

The aforementioned lack of awareness of others as distinct and separate from the Nagger can also lead to their perception and assumption that what you or others do or fail to do is a negative reflection on them. That is, they were not competent enough to ensure that you or others did what they wanted or were told to do. This perception can also play a role in their need to nag as their self-esteem is affected where you or others don't act in accord with their wishes or demands. Their unclear or enmeshed psychological boundaries with you and others can lead the Nagger to believe that others should promptly meet their spoken and/or unspoken demands, wishes, orders, and the like with no questions or no other alternatives offered. They know what needs to be done, and "You should just do it" can be their attitude.

The Nagger in your life may overly care about others' perceptions and approval. They can be seeking admiration and have other self-absorbed behaviors and characteristics where they look outside of themselves for validation, reassurance of their worth, and verification of their superiority. They may also not have a firm understanding that others are not extensions of them so that they take what you do and are as a reflection on them. This is a flawed perception and understanding that can lead them to think that if you don't live up to their standards, then others will think less of them and they will be shamed. They may think that they have the right and responsibility to nag you to do what they think is needed so that others will approve and think well of them.

Possible Strategies for Coping with the Nagger

The major and first set of coping strategies has to do with you, how you feel, and managing your feelings. This will be fundamental for implementing actions to better cope with the Nagger in your life. The primary strategies in the moment are:

Breathe—take calming breaths to control your negative feelings.

Accept that you are powerless to change them.

Use your emotional insulation to prevent catching their emotions *and* to prevent your frustration or other negative feeling from emerging and/or being acted on.

Present a neutral demeanor, facial expression, and body positioning. This also helps with your emotional insulating actions.

Avoid presenting negative reactions in the moment as this tends to increase their defensiveness about the correctness of what they are going or having to remind you to do. For example, don't mutter under your breath, roll your eyes, sigh, and the like.

Other self-management technique and strategies could be to hum and to visualize the Nagger as singing or dancing or as having a halo over their head or in a funny position. The visualization you choose can be anything that helps you in the moment to internally grin or chuckle. A humorous visualization gets you out of your negative reaction, which helps you better think about what to do and does not convey anything negative that the Nagger can discern and add to their grievance, feelings of being unappreciated, or that they are "right."

The use and effectiveness of the next set of strategies and techniques depend on the level and depth of the relationship you have with the Nagger in your life. That is, select a strategy or technique based on the value you have for the relationship. Trying some can help you decide which may be useful for you and those that do not fit you or the situation. When selecting or using a particular strategy or technique, it can be helpful to keep the following in mind. The Nagger can:

Feel misunderstood, unappreciated, and not valued

Provide more information and details than is warranted or needed

Think that your actions or inactions are a negative reflection on them

Adopt a long-suffering attitude

Be convinced that they do not need to change and that you and others do need to change

Be fearful of being perceived as inadequate

Let's term the following as trial-and-error strategies. When one does not work, try another one, but remember that what works at one time may not work at another time and vice versa. This is why you may need to memorize all of the suggestions.

Suggest that a partial accomplishment will be adequate (most times they will not agree).

Create a contact where they will post a list of what needs to be done *and* will not give you verbal reminders, explanations, or other embellishments.

Acknowledge that you recognize that they are trying to be helpful and that you are managing whatever it is.

Agree that you should remember.

Just accept that they are correct and don't argue.

Try a distraction for the moment.

Leave.

All of these suggestions are attempts to get the Nagger to shut up without using those specific words. Trying to negotiate doing just a part of what they want to be done might work for a major task that has many subtasks. However, they are likely to return to nagging about the rest so you've only quieted them for the moment. If you can get the Nagger to give you or post a list of what needs to be done or other reminders, that too can reduce their talking. This contract still has to be fulfilled on your part, but you don't have to listen to them or maybe catch their anxiety. Some gesture of appreciation for their diligence, although the way that they choose to do this is aggravating, can be welcomed by them. They may feel unappreciated, and this gesture can show that their efforts are noticed. The downside to using this strategy is that they can be encouraged, emboldened, and reinforced to continue nagging, or to even increase it. If their nagging is of concern and/or having a negative effort on the relationship, you would not want to do anything that encourages them to continue to nag.

For this particular moment, you could just agree with the Nagger that whatever it is needs to be done and, then follow through by doing it. Sometimes that may be sufficient. But don't worry, the Nagger is also very apt to find something else to nag about. Providing a distraction may work at times as this gets them off of the topic for which they are nagging. Distractions such as bringing their attention to a current problem or concern; pointing out something in the immediate environment that is a visual or auditory distraction; acting silly, humming, and remarking on the weather forecast; and the like could cease their nagging for the moment. The last suggestion is to leave their presence. Some way of leaving can be more palatable than are others:

Suddenly remember that you forgot something you need to take with you or to do and go to get or to do that

Look at the time and note that you need to leave, or you will be late, or to get gas or anything like that

Decide that you need to exercise

Take a bathroom break

There are numerous ways to leave. You may be able to think of more creative ways to leave their presence to get away from the nagging.

The techniques and strategies seem to suggest that any or all would be at best and marginally effective. The Nagger in your life is unlikely to change their need to nag because they see no need to change. They need their world to be in order and if they did not nag they would not get what they need. Their self-absorbed behavior and attitudes keep them focused on getting their needs met regardless of the negative consequences or impact on you, on the relationship or on others.

CHAPTER TEN

Reducing Your Stress and Anxiety

Introduction

The previous chapters addressed some of the possible reactions you can have in response to the anxious person in your life and presented some possible coping strategies. You have probably thought of some strategies that would better fit you personally and the anxious person. Also presented were descriptions for what your anxious person might be internally experiencing so as to help you better understand what may be fueling their anxiety, which then triggers their worry, complaints, micromanaging, or nagging. It is unlikely that you will be able to relieve their underlying anxiety or promote changes that will enable them to become less anxious. That is beyond your control and could be beyond their control. It can be important for your peace of mind to accept this and to not try to get them to change. This can be even more difficult for you to accept and live with if the relationship you have with the anxious person is close or intimate. Although it can be tempting to try to "fix" your anxious person, you will find it to be more constructive and helpful for both of you to work on yourself instead of the other person. This final chapter describes how you can be more helpful to them by being a model for calmness and steadiness, using thoughtful responding and reactions, and learning more effective actions, and how you can become better able to handle anxiety-producing situations. The first step is to reduce your stress, which then helps you reduce your anxiety.

Reduce Your Stress

One reason for the negative impact of the anxious person in your life has on you can be the stress you are under from other events, situations, relationships, and people in your life. You can be more susceptible to their emotional sending, less able to use your emotional insulation, less inclined to try to access techniques and strategies that work for you, and more open to catching their anxiety. This susceptibility along with your need to be helpful and/or to "fix it" can increase your stress and "make you feel crazy." It can feel like it is more than you can do to try and cope with at the time, especially when your anxious person seems to be constantly in crisis and coming to you to reduce their anxiety. There are two basic thoughts to recall when trying to cope with the anxious person in your life:

You are not responsible for their anxiety.

You cannot change them.

These thoughts can be somewhat stress reducing and calming when encountering your anxious person, and there are other general stress-reducing strategies and techniques you can use with them and others, and when events in your life produces stress for you. Let's take a look at some stress-reducing strategies.

Reducing Your Stress Helps You Cope

There are many benefits for reducing your stress: improving your health, clarifying your thoughts, containing your emotions and psychological well-being, promoting appreciation and pleasure in your life, building and fortifying your important relationships, achieving balance, and being an inspiration for others. You are encouraged to try the described activities for reducing stress, identify those that work best for you, and to create additional strategies and techniques. Also helpful is to keep a log or journal about the level of your stress at various times during a day, the stress-reducing activity(ies) you tried at that time, and if those activities were successful or not. You could categorize the success as none, little or moderate, or good. This would enable you to have a record that you could review periodically to be more aware of how you may be successfully managing your stress. Presented are simple activities for:

Eliminating some actions that have been shown to cause stress

Physical self-soothing techniques and activities

Cognitive self-soothing techniques and activities

Creative self-soothing techniques and activities

Relational self-soothing techniques and activities

Mood boosters and distractors

Finding your balance

Let's begin with having you think about your thoughts, actions, and other activities that could be causing you some stress that are under your control.

Your Actions That Contribute to Your Stress

You may be unaware of the thoughts, actions, and other activities you engage in that could be contributing to your stress and that you could reduce or eliminate. Read the following list and keep a mental check of all that you do every day or regularly. This list can get you thinking of other activities you could reduce or eliminate that would result in you feeling more in control and a greater sense of well-being, and allow you better control your anxiety and to cope with that for other people in your life.

Your long-term and short-term goals are murky. You aren't clear on what you want to be or do.

You feel unappreciated and that others do not recognize your contributions or worth.

The demands you place on yourself and on others are unrealistic, such as perfection.

Your associates tend to be like you and reinforce your depressing thoughts about the world.

You have excessive reliance on others for help, support, and affirmation of your value and worth.

You seldom or never engage in self-reflection, introspection, and critical self-examination.

You seem to constantly be irritable and/or angry.

You easily access your guilt and shame.

You expect favors from others and are constantly disappointed when these do not appear.

You tend to dither, ruminate, and obsess especially over trivial matters.

You keep doing the same thing that does not work, but you still expect different results and are constantly disappointed.

Your work, work space, and/or living space; car interior; thoughts; and the like tend to be and remain disorganized.

You do not let any distractions from your worry occur or get in the way of continually worrying about something.

Actions are mainly to please someone else and are not what would please you.

You panic frequently and don't know how to stop.

You worry about intangibles, events, or people who are not under your control.

You constantly look at or listen to the news.

You try to change another person.

You do not have any pastimes, hobbies, and the like that you could do daily.

You overindulge, such as eating, exercise, gambling, and drinking.

You frequently overcommit to do things.

You could decide to eliminate one of these a month, review how that worked for you, and then try to eliminate or reduce another one. In addition, you could begin to use one or more of the self-soothing activities described in the following sections and notice how that could be reducing your stress.

Physical Self-soothing Techniques and Strategies

Anxiety is felt in the body and usually produces tension that is felt in the muscles and other body parts, some of which may be below your level of awareness, such as your blood pressure.

Reflections: Take a moment here and do a body scan to see where tension is in your body. Begin with the top of your head, down through your neck, shoulders, arms, hands, chest, stomach, hips, thighs, legs, and ending at your feet. Did you notice tension in your body that was below your level of awareness? A technique you can try is to focus on the particular tension, such as your shoulders, consciously tense them more, hold for two to three seconds, and then release. Notice any difference, and maybe do the tensing again.

When high or acute, anxiety can cause a rapid heartbeat and pulse; a felt need to move the body, such as repetitive gestures like a foot jiggling; shallow breathing; and voice patterns such as rapid speech or talking loudly. Attending to and/or using some self-soothing physical activities can not only help you maintain your psychological balance and reduce and control your anxiety in general, but these can help you better cope with the anxious person in your life.

First, let's take inventory of your current physical self-soothing activities.

ACTIVITY 10.1 CURRENT PHYSICAL SELF-SOOTHERS

Materials: A sheet of paper and a writing instrument. If you usually work on a computer or table, this activity can be completed that way. Also, you will need a suitable working surface and a place to work that is free from disruptions or interruptions.

Procedure: Sit in silence and reflect on the physical self-soothers you use.

1. Divide the paper into four columns. Label the first column "Self-soothers categories," label the second column "Current activities," label the third column "Effectiveness," and label the fourth column "Needed Actions."

2. Under the column-labeled categories, write the following categories leaving sufficient space (about two to three inches) between each so that there is room to list category-related activities in the second column. The category

column should fill up the entire page. Categories are health patterns, movement, external body soothers, and body awareness.

3. Beside each category for column 1, list your current activities for each category. Examples for each category are:

Health patterns—sleep, nutrition, dental, checkups, and the like

Movement—exercise, dance, cleaning, yard work, yoga

External body soothers—massage, showering, slathering on lotion, soaking baths

Body awareness—breathing, location of tension, mindfulness, aches and pains

4. In column 3, give each activity you listed in column 2 an effectiveness rating from 0—not effective for you to 10—extremely effective.

5. Review your effectiveness ratings and put a checkmark beside activities that are rated 3 or below, and those that are rated 7 or above.

6. The final column is where you can decide on an action; plan to either increase your use of the most effective activities; and decrease, eliminate, or find a better activity to substitute for those rated 3 or below for their effectiveness. This can also be the time for you to reflect on the actions that are unhealthy, not useful, or even detrimental for you.

7. The final step involves reviewing what you wrote for the four columns and use the back of the sheet of paper to list the actions you want to decrease, those you want to decrease or eliminate, and new activities that you thought of as you completed the activities that could be constructive and useful.

A final caveat, don't try to make too many changes at the same time. Select those that are easiest to implement, and move from there to the most difficult or complex ones.

Two activities are presented to help you get started, breathing and a 10-minute decluttering process.

ACTIVITY 10.2 BREATHING

Find a comfortable place to practice breathing. The place should be free from disruptions and distractions such as sounds and sights that may get your attention and distract you. You can practice this process sitting or lying down. You may want to record the directions in advance, use soothing classical music or a recording of soothing sounds, and use a timer to sound a soft ting when your designated practice time is completed.

1. As you start the activity, notice your breathing, the tension spots, or aches or other places of discomfort in your body. Some people find that it is easier to concentrate on their breathing if their eyes are open, while others prefer to close their eyes. Either way will work.

2. Place your hand on your body where your breath seems to be coming from, such as the top of your chest, top of your stomach, or deeper down. Note if your breath is rapid or slow.

3. Consciously try to breathe deeper and slower. Notice what happens to the other parts of your body. Keep breathing as deeply and slowly as you can for as long as you set the timer for or a suitable period of time. Attempt to breathe slowly and deeply for five minutes. Practice as long as you can, and try to increase the number of minutes you breathe deeply and slowly each time you practice.

4. After each session, notice how your body feels and if the tension, aches, or places of discomfort have lessened. Some may even be eliminated, and some may remain unchanged. Try to focus on your overall feeling of well-being, relaxation, clarity of thoughts, as well as your physical sensations after each session.

Breathing can be done at any time and almost everywhere. Try consciously breathing as you ride in an elevator. When you are anxious or encounter the anxious person in your life, you can help resist catching their anxiety by trying to consciously breathe deeply and evenly as well as instituting your emotional insulation.

ACTIVITY 10.3 10-MINUTE DECLUTTERING

The act of decluttering can be both a physical self-soothing activity and a mental distraction. Used this way, it can help reduce some of your anxiety by moving your attention to something that is beneficial for you, can help clear your mind and thoughts, and will provide you with a more pleasing environment. Described here is a 10-minute procedure for decluttering your desk as an example. Other possible easily accessible decluttering spaces can be the following:
A drawer—desk drawer, in the kitchen or another room

Your purse or briefcase

Your e-mail and spam

One or more e-mail files

A room

A table, bookcase, or other piece of furniture

Decluttering a Desk

1. Remove books and shelve them; remove magazines and shelve them or put in the proper place.

2. Put pens and pencils in a holder or cup or where they can be easily accessed.

3. Start with the top sheets of paper or file folders on the desk and one by one as you encounter them:

    a. Either file promptly, or if you know you will have several pieces or documents for the same file, place them in a pile for filing all at one time

    b. Discard

    c. Place in a pile for prompt action.

4. Discard or put in drawers other items that are on the desk.

5. Work for 10 minutes and stop.

Take a breath, visually survey your desk or space, and notice how much more organized it is.

You may find that you too feel more organized. This decluttering procedure can be used for other spaces. Once you experience how much difference a 10-minute decluttering action can make, you can do that more often, which decreases the amount of clutter that can build up over time. And you can use some time to tackle the clutter in some of your other spaces. Try to notice your anxiety levels before and after you declutter a space.

Self-soothing—Cognitive

You may be able to reduce some of your anxiety by managing your thoughts about the situation that is producing the anxiety, the thoughts and apprehensions about your inner essential self, and tapping into a more valid reality. Rational Emotive Behavioral Therapy (REBT, Ellis) would propose that it isn't the event that triggers your anxiety; it is how you feel about the event. In the same way, how you feel about your inner essential self as being competent and able or doubting your competency to handle the situation could also be a contributor to your anxiety. Finally, how could you achieve a more valid and realistic perspective can be helpful.

You may be worried about something and thereby become anxious and find that it is difficult or impossible for you to not spend a considerable amount of time worrying, try to stop or distract yourself, but find that you continue to return to your worry over and over again. This is unproductive worry that wastes your time and energy and is unlikely to produce a viable outcome. In addition, this worry can cause you to be irritable and cranky, thereby impairing some of your relationships. These are two reasons to use some self-soothing cognitive strategies, and following are activities to get you started.

ACTIVITY 10.4 MANAGING THOUGHTS

Materials: A sheet of paper and a writing instrument, a suitable writing surface, and a place to work that is free from distractions and interruptions.
Procedure

1. Write a one- to two-word category or title for the concern or situation you are thinking about, such as financial, work-related, health, and the like.

2. Under that word or phrase, write the basic or essential thought you have about the concern in a short phrase, for example, financial—not enough income, mother's health—deteriorating.

3. List all of the feelings you experience during the time you think about your concern as you complete the activity, for example:

   Financial

   Not enough income

   Fearful, shame, guilt, anger

Try to list all of the feelings or even the thoughts about feelings, such as nervous, jittery, tense, and the like.

4. Copy each feeling you wrote in item # 3 as a list and make an association for yourself for that feeling. Some examples for possible associations are incompetent, inadequate, not good enough, a failure, not treated fairly, exploited, and so on.

5. Once you have your list of self-associations, sit for a moment and reflect on the validity of each association. Then give each association a validity rating of 0—no validity, 1—a little validity, 2—fair validity, 3—adequate validity, 4—very valid, or 5—extremely valid.

6. Put a checkmark beside each association that has a validity rating of 3 or above. Review these and see if any of the ratings need adjustment. For example, you may have rated a current self-association as 4, but, upon reflection, you could now rate it as 2 or lower. The concern hasn't changed, but your associations with the concern about yourself may have become more balanced and realistic. This change could allow you to think more clearly about possible actions, solutions, or moderating your expectations of yourself.

The previous activity guided you to start considering the validity of some of your thoughts about yourself. The next activity assists you in awareness of positive thoughts about yourself.

ACTIVITY 10.5 MY THOUGHTS ABOUT MYSELF

Materials: A sheet of paper, a writing instrument, a suitable writing surface, and a suitable place to work that is free from interruptions and disruptions.
Procedure

1. List the following down one side of the paper leaving room to write beside each: Major Interests, Major accomplishments, Talents/abilities, Wishes for myself, and Pleasurable activities.

2. Now, list three to five things about yourself beside each item that relates to you or describes you. For example: Major Interests: Reading, Writing Teaching, Research Major Accomplishments: Publishing, Promotion, Organizational President.

3. Review your lists, note your feelings as you write and review, and then write a summary statement about the thoughts you have about yourself.

Creative Self-soothing Strategies

Using creative activities as self-soothers can be helpful even if you don't think of yourself as being creative. Creative, as used here, means engaging in a new or novel process or procedure. Examples of possible areas for being creative include cooking; landscaping; decorating; streamlining a complex issue, problem, or concern; learning a new fun task such as magic tricks; and trying different uses for ordinary items. Opportunities to be creative are all around and do not always require specialized training or talent. Creative self-soothers can also be art; writing; music such as singing, dancing, performing, or other musical activities; crafts such as fiber arts, knotting, and crocheting; and any other creative activity that distract and enrich as well as is soothing. Following are some ideas in Activity 10.6 to get you start thinking about possibilities for your creative self-soothers.

Relational Self-soothers

So far, all of the proposed possible self-soothers are focused on you. However, it can be soothing for some people to focus some attention on others as avenues for soothers, especially if what you do is to be altruistic where you give of yourself without any expectations of reciprocity. Doing so is altruistic and not in response to the other person's demands or requests although what you do could fulfill a need of theirs. The anxious

---

ACTIVITY 10.6 CREATIVE EXTENSIONS FOR COMMON THINGS

Materials: You will need paper and a writing instrument to compile your ideas. After which you will need to appropriate materials to try out the idea from your list.
Procedure

1. List 5–10 ideas for different versions or uses for the following. One example possibility is listed for each.

    Grilled cheese sandwich: with sliced apple

    Newspaper—tear or cut a heart shape and post on a card or a sheet of paper or in an old book

    Wrapping paper—tear to use as a background for a collage

    Old worn gloves, or scarf, or another article of clothing: arrange the item on a sturdy background such as card stock, write or print a description of it or a poem or a cinquain about the article, paste or glue on poster board and put in a frame

    Knit, crochet, or sew: make a set of placemats for your table

    Scrapbook: arrange pages of pictures or artifacts for a holiday, or a trip, or a project you are planning.

2. Review your lists, select one to complete and follow through. As you gather the materials for the activity and complete it, notice how you think and feel during the activity, and how you feel after you complete it. Notice if you are less tense or anxious.

You can find that you can think of many more creative self-soothing activities that are pleasurable as well as reduce some of your anxiety.

person in your life can be so draining of your time, energy, and other things such as resources, and you are having to respond to them so much that you overlook others in your world, not totally, but to a point where they can feel neglected. Since you are a helper (notice that to always or almost always respond or attend to the anxious person in your life), you may find it soothing at times to relate to or connect with others as a source for soothing. If you already do some of the suggested actions that follow, and these are satisfying for you, it can be beneficial for you to increase these actions. There may also be some suggestions that you can try to see if they provide solace and are soothing.

Practice giving someone one act of kindness every day.

Volunteer for a charity such as the local foodbank.

Smile at a child or a person in a wheelchair.

Write a positive note to a loved one and place it where it will be a surprise for them.

Help a child with homework.

Mow or rake the lawn for an elderly neighbor.

Smile and say "Good morning" to people you meet.

Tell someone something you appreciate about them.

Send a "sweet tweet" to someone you haven't talked with in a while.

Listen to a child or a teen or a shut-in for 15 minutes free from any distractions such as phone or television.

You can probably think of many more relational acts that could be self-soothers for you.

Mood Triggers and Boosters

Take a moment to reflect on what your mood is when you are not or are less anxious, more confident and feel more in control. Our moods affect our ability to problem solve, make decisions, relate to others, and our connections to ourselves and to the larger universe. Although moods tend to be transitory, can change rapidly, and are influential for our thoughts, behaviors, attitudes, and feelings, they are also responsive to our conscious interventions to change them.

Reflection: Think of a time—day, week, or hour—where you were grumpy or blue. Can you identify what changed you from being grumpy or blue? Can you recall how you felt and acted after you came out of that mood? Was there something that happened to you that contributed to the mood change?

Situations, people, and our and other's actions can trigger our moods whether the mood is positive or negative. Some terms that signal a negative mood are as follows:

Blue—down, deflated, depressed

Grumpy—irritable, touchy, hypersensitive

Antsy—tense, edgy, apprehensive

Aggressive—fighting, sensitive

Terms associated with a positive mood can be similar to the following:

Walking on air—happy, cheerful

In the mood for love—appreciated, connected to others

Upbeat—see possibilities, good anticipations

All's right with the world—pleasant, comfortable, in control

There may be times when life circumstances seem to produce a mood where everything seems hopeless and you feel helpless. For example, your or a loved one's illness can contribute to a negative mood. Or, when it seems as if nothing in your world is going right or as you hoped it would. Or, you are anticipating something dire, and other similar situations. It is situations like these that contribute to our moods and to our anxiety.

You can help reduce your anxiety by boosting your mood as it is difficult to be anxious when your mood is positive. You may not have thought about changing your mood as a tactic to decrease your anxiety, but you may want to try some mood boosters and see what the impact is on your thinking, feeling, and actions.

Your Mood Triggers

There is a process that leads you to developing a mood that has both conscious and unconscious factors. This process is illustrated as follows:

Triggers Occur

these lead to

Negative Thoughts about your self

which lead to

Negative Feelings about your self

these collect and Become a

Mood

Mood triggers are unique to the individual and are usually a combination of factors including current and former live events; chance of happenings; the weather; current physical, cognitive, and emotional states and well-being; internal and external demands and expectations; and so on. These are explored further later in this section. The important point about triggers is that these can lead to negative thoughts about oneself.

What seems to trigger negative moods for you? Some possibilities can include the following:

- Gloomy weather
- Feeling shut in
- Feeling alienated or isolated
- Having a bad day where nothing seems to go right
- Being disappointed
- Illness
- Not getting your way
- Someone criticizing, blaming, or chastising you

Identifying the trigger(s) for your negative mood can suggest some possible actions that you can take to get out of the negative mood or to prevent it. Actions such as prior preparation, avoidance, and distractions could be possibilities. But this is just the beginning. Not having a negative mood is preferable, and you may be able to reduce or eliminate some triggers for yourself. But, on the other hand, taking action to boost your mood can also be helpful, especially when you find that you are anxious.

Mood Boosters

Mood boosters are the thoughts and actions you can implement that have demonstrated effectiveness for you, and you may even create some

Activity 10.7 My Mood Trigger(s)

Materials: Sheets of paper and a pen or pencil or a suitable digital device.
Procedure

1. Gather materials and find a place to work with a suitable working surface free from intrusions and disruptions or distractions.
2. Begin with an awareness of your present mood and record this with either a word or phrase.
3. If your mood is positive, record your feelings at this time. Then recall your most recent negative mood and the feelings that accompanied that mood.
4. If your mood is negative at this time, record the feelings you are experiencing.
5. Use either the negative mood in Step 4 or 5 and try to identify when the negative mood began. Record your answers to as many of the following as possible:

    *   What day of the week, time of day, and/or time of year did you become aware of the mood?
    *   What were you doing, and what were you feeling about yourself?
    *   Who was present, or were you alone?
    *   Identify three activities you did prior to the mood.
    *   How satisfied were you with your life overall at that time?

6. Review the answers you wrote for Step 5 and determine if there was a feeling, thought, action, or person(s) that was the defining point for your negative mood. For example, you may have received bad news, and appliance may have needed repairs; you clashed with a peer or family member, or the mood just seemed to appear out of nowhere.
7. If you did identify one or more triggers, now think back over a longer period of time and recall if something similar triggered prior negative moods.
8. If you could not identify a specific trigger, continue to try to identify what triggered your mood. For example, can you recall what events were happening to and around you at that time? There could be a collection of events that caused the triggered mood. Or, were you ruminating about your satisfaction with yourself, your achievements, and the like? Or, were you thinking about your failures, lost opportunities, lack of options or alternatives, or fear of possible future events?
9. If you have some ideas about your trigger(s), record these.

possible new ones. There are some assumptions about using mood boosters.

- Mood boosters are individual and personal.
- Your understanding of your wants, needs, and desires guides you in the selection of boosters.
- You have many aspects of your essential inner self, and each aspect has several alternatives for boosters.
- Selecting and using your boosters can be facilitated by self-observation of some of your behavior patterns.
- There can be some self-imposed barriers and constraints.
- Boosters do not have to be costly.

No one mood booster fits everyone. You are a unique individual, and what works for you may not work for others. And what works for you at a particular time and place in your life may not work when you are in another place and time. You are encouraged to consider each of the categories of boosters that follow and how they may apply to you. You may even want to try some that initially do not seem to be appealing to you. Make your own choices.

It can be easy to think of something exciting and interesting that will boost your mood and is costly. Or, while that booster may be soothing in the short term it may not or will not be good for you in the long term. Activities like many of the following may seem attractive, but can carry unpleasant consequences for the long term.

- Shopping especially if you overspend
- Alcohol use
- Mood-altering substances
- Overeating
- Eating junk food to excess
- Gambling when you cannot afford to lose
- Excessive exercise
- Engaging in out-of-control or risky sexual behavior
- Gaming such as video games

There are less costly and more effective ways to lift your mood.

Low-cost Mood Boosters

Low- or no-cost mood boosters can be found in many aspects of your life. For example, there are sensory, cognitive, relational, creative, and physical categories, and each of these has many actions and techniques that you can use.

Sensory—This category refers to boosting your mood through one or more of your senses: visual, auditory, smell, taste, and tactile.

What do you see that boosts your mood? What sounds, such as music, boost your mood? Are there smells that make you smile, or are pleasing? Think of the tastes that are pleasing, are satisfying, and wake up your taste buds. What soothes your skin, for example, a silk shirt? Can you find some of these in your world that are either low or no cost?

Cognitive—This category includes actions related to your mental functioning such as thought stopping, self-affirmation, and use of your imagination.

Does it boost your mood to think about a pleasant anticipated event, or to remember a past one? Can you stop self-denigrating thoughts and focus on your assets? Can you imagine succeeding at something almost impossible to achieve?

Relational—This category focuses on the lift you can gain from others in your world such as your altruistic acts toward others, appreciation for what your loved ones give to you, and awareness of the impact of your moods on them.

Try making a gratitude tree. Cut or tear five to six strips of paper in graduated strips with different lengths. Then, write something you are thankful for on each strip. Paste the strips on a piece of cardstock beginning about 2" from the bottom using the longest strip first, and then pasting the strips in graduated lengths. Cut or tear a 1–1 ½" strip for the trunk of the tree. Draw a small heart at the top of the tree.

Creative—This is the category for engaging in creative activities where the process allows you to move away from thoughts, feelings, and ideas that may be causing distress, and to move toward immersing yourself in acts that produce a product and greater satisfaction with your essential inner self.

Try a new recipe, or craft, or return to an old craft. Make something you like such as a collage or a drawing, or write a poem.

Physical—This category contains bodily actions and movements that you can take to lift your mood, are healthy, and do not cause distress for anyone else.

Skip down the pathway. Whirl around as you did when you were a child and did this for no reason. Take a new exercise class or video. Dance when no one is watching.

Building a More Effective Inner Self

In addition to reducing your stress and anxiety, you can reflect on how to build a more effective inner self. The self-psychologists call this healthy adult narcissism, which is a goal worth striving for. It means that you will have a healthy self-focus when needed, that the more destructive aspects of self-absorbed behaviors and attitudes are moderated, and that you are more accepting of yourself and of others.

A healthier and more effective inner essential self begins with a focus on healthy adult narcissism. Why focus on healthy adult narcissism? Reasons for such a focus are to understand the behaviors and attitudes that are affirming to your self-esteem, provide guidance for building more enduring and satisfying relationships, fortify you so as to better cope with the anxious person in your life, and assist you to be a model for them as encouragement to become more effective. The characteristics that will be briefly described are empathy, wisdom, zest, appreciation for beauty and wonder, and altruism.

Empathy was discussed in more detail earlier in the book The description here uses the same definition phrased as a capacity to enter the experiencing of the other person and to feel what that person is feeling without losing the sense of oneself as being separate and distinct from the person. It can be very validating and affirming to be understood deeply when you receive empathy, and the capacity to be empathic strengthens relationships as well as provides comfort to the other person.

It is important to note that empathy is most effective when openly and directly expressed to that person. Most helpful is to identify and name the feeling the other person is experiencing, such as apprehension, anger, or embarrassment. Empathic responding is not sympathy, conveyed nonverbally, or saying something like "I understand." Although any of these responses may be helpful, it is important to understand that they are not empathic responses.

Wisdom is developed over time as you learn from your experiences, learn from others' experiences, can apply critical thinking to form your opinions and decisions that are open to older-natives and new knowledge without losing your core values, and live and act in accord with your core values. Wisdom is characterized by actions and attitude such as the following:

The ability to moderate and curb impulses

Manage and contain intense emotions especially negative ones such as anger and resentment

The capacity to stay focused on meaningful priorities every day and for the long term

Identify what is important and significant, and what is not

Understand and accept the limits of personal power and control

Evaluate when to persevere

Judge when the forces and resistances are unable to be overcome

Work through adversity when needed but do not seek it out

Have balance in your life

Not doing the same thing that does not work and continuing to expect a different outcome

Wisdom is not easily obtained but is very valuable for a rich and rewarding life.

Zest can be described as having enthusiasm, energy, and excitement, whether these be for work, life, relationships, an avocation, or a cause. There are many aspects of life where zest can be focused and realized. Ask yourself what energizes, interests, and captures your attention. You could have zest for any of the following:

Engaging in recreation or sports activities

Working for a cause such as combating hunger

Creative activities such as art, music, dance, and performing

Learning in any area, be that cooking, gardening, academic pursuits, history, and so on

Helping others by volunteering for community agencies and the like

Teaching people to read

Video games and gaming

Where do you put your enthusiasm? How do you feel after participating or engaging in a pursuit where you have zest? My hunch is that your spirits are lifted, you have an increased sense of well-being, and you are better able to do those things that contribute positively to your life.

Beauty and wonder are all around us and make positive contributions to our lives when we can take time to notice and appreciate them. Each of us may have a different perception of what we consider as beauty and wonder. The important thing is not to agree on what constitutes beauty and/or wonder; it is just that it is helpful for our sense of meaning, purpose, and well-being to appreciate them when they do appear in our lives.

Appreciating beauty and wonder can lift our spirits; provide inspiration; enhance the feeling of well-being and, as being connected to the universe and to others, give us calming and serene moments; contribute to moments of happiness; encourage and support us in our times of despair or adversity; and contribute to hope and many other positives for us.

Altruism can be conceptualized as giving of our self to others without expecting reciprocity. What is given is done so freely purely for the benefit of the receiver and is truly a gift. Such altruistic acts do not have to be monumental or major; they can be simple everyday kindness as well as those that call for extensive efforts on your part. Let's try and think of some altruistic acts you and others may have received.

The medical personnel who stayed beyond office hours to take care of your medical needs

Providing school materials for children in need

Visiting and talking with a shut in

Offering to babysit so a single parent or the spouse of a deployed military parent could have an afternoon out

Coaching a child's sports team

A teacher remaining after school to help a struggling student

Cutting the lawn for a sick or elderly person

Changing a tire for a stranger on the road

Remaining with someone who is ill or hurt until the emergency personnel arrive

Understanding and responding to someone who is despondent

You can probably think of more examples as there are many altruistic acts extended every day.

The final part of the chapter focuses on prevention strategies for negative thoughts, feelings, and moods that can emerge in interactions with the anxious person in your life. You are encouraged to create, develop, and recall some actions and thoughts that can be used as prevention. Suggested prevention strategies and techniques are in the following categories:

- Acceptance of personal limitations
- Daily attention to fortifiers
- Retreats, happy places, and sanctuaries
- Happy moments
- Self-care

Preventive strategies emphasize building and fortifying your essential inner self so that when negative events and situations occur, you do not allow yourself to become affected to the point where you get and keep a negative mood. Yes, negative things do happen, but your reactions to these may be more about you and how you feel about your essential inner self than the negative events and situations themselves.

Accept Your Limitations

Knowing, understanding, and accepting your limitations lead to wisdom, a reduction of grandiosity, and a more realistic self-appraisal, all of which are to be cultivated and that can be enriching of your life. There are limits on what you can control and on your responsibilities, but you may not have reflected on this before in a systematic way. Consider if any of the following thoughts, feelings, and actions are reflective of you.

- It's my responsibility to take care of the emotional well-being of other adults who are able to care for themselves.
- I have to ensure that everything goes well for others.
- If someone is distressed or upset, I must take care of what is causing the distress and also soothe them.
- I get very upset when things don't go as planned and feel that it is my fault.

- Others will not like or love me unless I can always meet their needs.
- I should not ever do or say anything that upsets or disappoints another person.
- I am responsible for others' feelings.
- Bad things will happen if I don't take care of everything.

Other such thoughts, attitudes, and convictions also point to an inability to accept one's personal limitations. Take a look at the list and reflect on how unrealistic it is to believe that only you are responsible for an outcome, that your actions or lack of actions are so important and powerful, or that you alone have these obligations. Also reflect on how many times you could not live up to these unrealistic self-imposed expectations. You can increase your awareness of these and try to eliminate them. It could also be helpful for you to work to understand how you are making unrealistic demands and expectations on yourself and to become more realistic.

There are some short-term suggestions that may help.

- Recognize and accept that competent adults are responsible for their welfare. You may be able to help them at times, but they bear the major responsibility for their welfare as you do for yours.
- Remember that you can choose your feelings about yourself and resolve to have more positive ones, fewer negative ones, and less intense negative feelings. For example, you can feel regretful instead of the more intense guilty.
- Just as you can choose your feelings, so can others. You are not powerful enough to cause others' feelings. You may say or do something that related to triggering these for another person, but they are in charge of their feelings, not you. You can make *a* difference, but, in most cases, you do not make *the* difference. Recognize and accept that your contribution may be important, but it is most likely not critical.

Becoming more realistic about this can be a powerful preventive tool.

Give Daily Attention to Your Fortifiers

Don't wait until you feel down or experience a negative mood to pay attention to your fortifiers, those things that boost your mood and fortify your self-esteem. Instead, develop a habit of seeking out of positive in your life and doing so every day.

You have your own unique set of fortifiers, those things, actions, events, and the like that provide you with the spirit, hope, and assurances that can and will survive and thrive. You may not be fully aware of these and tap into their power every day, but you do have them although some may be dormant, not thought of, or need to be developed.

Reflection: What gets your day started? Do you seek out anything that helps you get your day moving well? Is there anything throughout the day that keep you in good spirits? What about your evening and night?

You probably thought of many possible fortifiers and may have realized that you do not tend to use or attend to these daily although they are readily at hand. Following are some possible and available fortifiers put into time categories: Getting the day started on a positive note, during the day, and evening possibilities. These, of course, may not fall neatly into time frames that fit for you, and some will not fit you or your lifestyle. These are examples presented to get you thinking about what your fortifiers are and how you can attend to them daily.

Starting the Day (Some can be done at any time of the day)

Music, energetic or soothing	Hugs from loved ones
Meditation	Exercising
Prayer	Seeing the sun rise
Religious readings	Having a good breakfast
Yoga or something similar	Getting off to work without forgetting
Taking a walk or running	anything important
Playing with a pet or a child	

During the Day

Giving and receiving smiles	Making appreciative comments
Finding something of beauty in the environment	Pleasant conversation
Dancing to the music	Practicing a move
Decluttering (workspace, home)	Stretching
Reading (magazine, book, etc.)	Taking a stroll

Evening

Use the relaxing and calming fortifiers from your morning, such as meditation or yoga

Work on your hobby and develop one if you do not have one at this time

Participate in a recreational activity

Get ready for the next day

Watch something interesting on television

Listen to music

Retreats, Happy Places, and Sanctuaries

Retreats, happy places, and sanctuaries are places where you can go to restore your essential inner self, to become centered and grounded, obtain serenity, and/or to examine your inner self and its resources. The places referred to here are either real or can be an imagined one. The idea is that when a negative mood creeps up on you, one tactic is to visualize your favorite retreat, happy place, or sanctuary and spend some time there if only for a few minutes. But, first, let's see what your place looks like.

ACTIVITY 10.8 MY SPECIAL PLACE

Directions are provided for three different ways to complete the exercise and a list of materials for each. Choose the method you feel best suits you.

Materials: Drawing—a sheet of paper and a set of colored pencils or felt markers, or crayons and a pen or pencil for writing.

Writing—A sheet of paper and a pen or pencil or a suitable digital device.

Photo—A photo of a place that gives you the feeling of a retreat or happy place or sanctuary, a sheet of paper, double-sided tape, and a pen or pencil. Or, if the suitable computer and software devices are available, the photo and exploration can be completed using these.

Procedure:

1. Read the first two steps before beginning to work. Gather materials and find a suitable place to complete the exercise that is free from distractions and interruptions.

2. Close your eyes, sit in silence, and try to clear your mind. Let an image of a place or setting emerge that gives you a feeling of being safe, pleased, and nurtured. Stay with that image as long as you like, noticing as many details of the image as you can such as colors, sounds, shapes, actions, and objects.

3. When you are ready, open your eyes and do one of the following.

    For drawing: Draw the place or setting.

    For writing: Write a complete description of your image.

    For the photo: Use the double-sided tape and tape the photo to the paper and write the details you recall when you closed your eyes.

    If you are working on the computer, use the software to paste the photo on a page and follow the photo directions in Step 3.

4. Next, make a list of the feelings evoked as you imaged your retreat, happy place or sanctuary, as you wrote or drew or on the computer, and now as you look at your product.

You now have an image that you can access whenever you feel a negative mood emerging or when you realize that one is getting worse. Just a brief respite can be enough to boost the mood.

Happy Moments

Few, if any, people can be happy all of the time, but all of us can experience happy moments. What is proposed here is that you begin to collect some happy moments to return to when you have the blues, blahs, or feel down in the dump.

Happy moments lift spirits, provide hope, increase feelings of physical well-being and has other such positive benefits. Like moods, these moments are usually brief and transitory although we may wish them to be more lasting and have sustainability. Prevention and intervention of your negative moods can be enhanced when you have and revisit some happy moments.

What can constitute a happy moment for you?

-   An unexpected recognition of an accomplishment
-   Being present when a family member does something important or makes him/her happy such as a birth, wedding, or receiving a sport or academic award.
-   When your solution to a problem works or produces a positive result.
-   Hearing that you did get the job, raise or promotion.
-   Being recruited for membership in something you want or feel is important.
-   Seeing your creative product on display.

- Finishing a complex, long involved project.
- A gift from someone significant to you.
- Playing
- The realization that you are getting better, recovering, or growing.
- Feeling at peace with yourself.

No one but you can define your happy moments and these are just suggestions to get you started thinking about what gives you the feeling of happiness if only for that moment or a short period of time.

Reflection: What do you do when you are happy: smile, twirl, dance, sing, whistle, and the like? When was the last time you did any of these or had a happy moment?

Self-care

The most effective prevention strategy is self-care where you attend to the various aspects of your life, try to make these as strong and viable as they can possibly be, and continue to grow and develop them. While there may be times when external events and situations need more of your attention, it is still important that you do not lose sight of the need to also take care of yourself.

Let's put self-care into the categories of physical, cognitive, relational, inspirational, creative and emotional.

Physical—the body and maintenance of its optional functioning.

Cognitive—your thoughts and ideas, and the clarity, logic and reasonableness of these

Relational—initiation and maintenance of satisfying, enduring and meaningful relationships

Inspirational—the meaning and purpose for your life

Creative—your flexibility and willingness to take a new or novel approach, assume new perspectives, and to produce new and novel products

Emotional—maintaining access to a variety of emotions, an ability to not get mired or bogged down in intense negative feelings, appropriate expressions for feelings, and the facility to manage and contain intense emotions.

Each of these categories of aspects of your self has numerous components and you may benefit at this point to consider where you are for each of these categories, to identify the components for each that are working well for you, and also identify the components that may need your attention for better or more optimal functioning.

Summary

This final chapter focused on prevention strategies that can keep you from getting mired in a negative mood when one emerges. Although what you developed as your personal strategies may not prevent you from having a down mood, these can and will fortify you so that your negative mood is of shorter duration. Make good use of what you have learned about yourself and about the anxious person in your life. You will be a help to yourself and to them. Good luck.

Tips and Hints: Mood Boosters, Effective Communications, Stress Reduction, and Creavitity[1]

10 Tips for Finding a Low- or No-cost Daily Mood Booster

What gets you down, grumpy, blue, or in an unpleasant mood? Although you may not be depressed, the mood may lead you into a downward descent that will result in sustained gloom; depression; feelings of being helpless, hopeless, or inadequate; or other such deflating thoughts and feelings. However, you do not have to get caught up in negative thoughts and feelings as it is possible to change your mood. There can be simple, quick, and low- or no-cost actions you can initiate to lift your spirits and banish a negative mood. You can change your reactions to having a negative mood.

Let's start with some of my favorite tips for finding a mood booster. After that are presented some additional actions to get you started on thinking and creating your own set of personal mood boosters.

Tips

1. Laugh out loud. Don't just smile; let go with a big belly laugh. Where can you find something funny? Try reading the comic strips, hearing or telling jokes, seeing something silly, or looking at animal antics on the internet.

---

1. Some of the material appeared in the author's blog on *Psychology Today*.

2. Whenever you could use a hug, reach out to someone you love and be affectionate—hug them, say appreciative things to someone, and give someone a compliment.

3. Smile at someone you do not know who may not usually receive a smile—at a child, a cashier, toll collector, and the like.

4. Pay attention to how something feels on your skin such as water on skin in the shower, a massage, or a lotion or cream as you smooth it on.

5. Seek out a pleasant aroma. For example, think of how a bakery smells, walk through a florist shop, smell perfume if you are not allergic, or think of how clean laundry smells.

6. Declutter and organize something small: purse, drawer, shelf, magazines, desk, or personal papers. Large decluttering projects can seem overwhelming and time consuming, so start small. For example, what can you do in 10 minutes to neaten a space such as a drawer?

7. Do something different—break a routine. Ideas can include driving a different route to the store or work, visiting a display of some kind, or checking out a farmer's market.

8. Perform a kind act. Look around and see how you may be able to perform an act of kindness.

9. Take a walk and notice your surroundings. Practice mindfulness, notice scents, sounds, colors, movements, pleasant visuals, and the like.

10. Bring some color into your life. For example, put a flower (real, silk, paper) or plant in a vase for your living or working space, set a container of colorful marbles or strips of paper where you can easily see it, or display fruit.

Try one of these each day for a week and notice the effect(s) on your mood.

10 Tips for More Effective Verbal Communications

You may be an excellent communicator and do not need tips to be more effective. In that case, I'm recommending that you read the following tips in case you have to give some tips to another person.

1. Don't provide too much information, background, context, and other details. Get to the main point early in the conversation. The other person does not have to know all of the information that you do in order to understand what you are talking about. You can always ask them if they need more information.

2. Provide only relevant information. Try to ensure that you provide only sufficient and necessary information so that the other person can understand what you are trying to communicate. They really need only the facts, not your speculations or fantasies. They are more likely to understand when you limit your communication to relevant information.

3. Be succinct and precise and focus on essentials. Too many words and concepts will be confusing. Remember that they are coming in at the middle of your thoughts, as you have been with whatever it is much longer than they have.

4. Listen to the other person and answer or respond directly to what they are saying or asking—not what you think is needed or meant. You may want to practice paraphrasing what another person says before adding your comment or asking questions. By paraphrasing you are letting the other person know what you understood them to be saying, and if there are errors in what you thought you heard, these can be more easily corrected.

5. Remember that too much information can be confusing to the other person. Think about how you feel when someone asks you several questions at the same time. You don't know which is most important, which to answer first, or what information they are seeking. The same is true when you give too much information at one time; the other person does not know what to focus on or what is most important for you.

6. Do not give details about other people, your rejected ideas and thoughts, musings, and the like. For example, when trying to convey some information about another person, it isn't helpful to the receiver to know details about that person that are not relevant to your message, such as how you came to know them and the different jobs they've held. It is also not very helpful to the listener to hear what you thought about and then rejected much less the reasons for your rejection. If these are helpful and relevant, let the listener ask for these details.

7. Do not change topics in midstream as that makes it difficult for anyone to follow your point(s). For example, let's say you were talking about the fall weather, and in the middle of your sentence, you switched to talking about how you suffer in the summer, or something similar—which are they supposed to respond to, the fall weather or your suffering in the summer. This is a simple example, and just think how confused the listener is when the topic is more complex, and you switch topics.

8. Talking about how you arrived at this point may not be relevant. Some people seem to need to give their life stories as prelude to getting to the current point, issue, or problem. This may be important information for them but probably does not add to the other person's understanding of your message or point.

9. Be judicious when talking about your feelings as not everyone is comfortable talking about feelings. Also, sometimes there is an implied message that you want the other person to take care of your feelings or do something

about them. That may not be your intent, but make sure you discuss your feelings with receptive people such as those who are close to you.

10. Give the other person time and space to express their thoughts, feelings, and ideas.

10 Tips for Immediate (or Almost Immediate) Stress Reduction

Stress in a constant given. Life produces stress, some of which is out of our control, and some can be controlled or even eliminated. Think of stress as an accumulation of small and large stressors that add up to produce BIG STRESS. Big stress gives us the feeling of being overwhelmed and able to cope or function as well as we would like.

I want to introduce the idea that some of your stress is self-induced, self-inflicted, and self-defeating. These are some of the behaviors and attitudes that can produce stress that are under your control and that you can reduce or eliminate. As you read these, reflect on how or if they fit you, and how you could relinquish it or them.

1. You may have murky goals so that you do not know what your priorities are or can work to achieve your goal(s). Start setting short-term or even daily goals and have a specific long-term realistic goal. It is also helpful to develop strategies to attain your goal.

2. Do you feel unappreciated? Are you using your time trying to get that appreciation, but mostly not succeeding? If feeling appreciated is important for you, try being kind, performing altruistic acts, and showing appreciation to those nearest and dearest to you.

3. It is very stressful to try to live by unrealistic standards and demands for yourself and/or for others, such as trying to achieve perfection. Take a moment to reflect on your standards and demands of yourself and others and gauge how realistic these may be. If they are not realistic, this may be causing stress because they are not attainable. Try being content with "good enough" for some things at some times, and see if that helps.

4. If you associate only with people you want to emulate and are using your time and effort trying to meet their expectations and values, you may find it less stressful to just meet your values and expectations. You may also want to expand your social support system to be more diverse.

5. Do not excessively rely on others for help, support, affirmation, and other things that you could do for yourself. Try to be as independent as possible.

6. Do not avoid self-reflection, introspection, and critical self-examination. When you resist this can produce stress. You may avoid these actions

because you fear what you may then know about yourself and not like it. Some self-reflection, introspection, and critical self-examination can be affirming of yourself, bring clarity, and suggest priorities and goals.

7. When you become angry or irritated and find it difficult to relinquish the feeling, that produces continued stress that affects your thinking, your body, your relationships, and your general sense of well-being. You can let go of negative feelings if you want to.

8. If you easily tap into your guilt and/or shame and find that this happens frequently, then you may find it less stressful to live and act in accord with your values and to work to better understand the roots of your guilt and shame and what triggers these for you.

9. If you expect favors from others, but are often disappointed, your disappointment is more about you than it is about the other person. See # 3.

10. Tend to dither, ruminate, or obsess over even trivial or minor things. Resolve to become more decisive and active. Just getting it done can be relieving and also save you time.

The tips presented actions that are under your control as they are your thoughts and feelings, most about yourself, and not about outside factors not under your control. It could be helpful to try one or two of the tips per week, evaluate their efficacy for you, and reflect on how you feel after trying them. Then, for the next week, continue what you started the previous week and add an additional one or two to try.

11 More Tips to Reduce Your Stress

Read through the following list to determine if any of these fit you, if they are causing you even minor stress, and how you might act differently so that you are not contributing to your stress. There are enough other things in your life that are stressful without you adding to your own distress.

1. If there is something in your life that you have and are trying to make better, to solve, or to help another person, reflect on what you are doing. Do you keep doing the same thing that has not worked, but you continue to do it expecting different results and find that you are continually disappointed? If so, you may want to think about not doing what is not working and see what happens. You can always think of something different to do that may have a better chance of working.

2. Look around you at this moment, visualize some of your other spaces, and note what you see. Do you keep your spaces disorganized? Spaces that

include your work space, living space, car interior, a purse or briefcase, and thoughts? Take some time and declutter one or more spaces and see how you feel. You may want to resolve to declutter something every day. Take 10 minutes and see how much you can accomplish.

3. When you worry do you let any distractions get in the way of your worrying? Do you find that you continually return to the issue, problem, or concern and worry? If so, you may want to develop a list of distractions that will take you away from the issue, problem, or concern as worrying about it isn't producing any solutions. Make yourself a list of distractors: visual such as window shopping or going to a movie; auditory such as listening to music or an inspirational audio message; movement such as walking or dancing; writing such as making lists or a journal entry; or anything that can serve as a distractor for the time being.

4. It can be very stressful to work mostly to please someone else instead of doing what you want. Yes, there are times when you do want to please someone, but if most of your time and effort is focused on pleasing that other person, you are contributing to your stress especially if it seems that they can never be satisfied.

5. Do you find that you panic quite often? Panic itself is very stressful and debilitating to your mind and body. It is not unusual to panic at times; there are even times when panic is the best reaction for you, but frequent panic is not. That is something you may want to work on with a competent and trained mental health professional. For the short term, when you panic it is helpful to breathe deeply, which is a calming technique. It may be difficult to do when you are panicking, but remind yourself that breathing will help and continue to make your breaths deep and as even as possible.

6. If you find that you worry about intangibles and events or people who are not under your control, you may be similar to the anxious person discussed in this book. Some of the suggestions provided for the Worrier may also be helpful for you.

7. There are people who constantly look at or listen to the news, and studies have shown that they are more distressed, stressed, upset, and less happy than people who either do not listen to the news or restrict their news intake. You may want to try limiting your attention to the news to reading the newspaper and listening to newscasts maybe once a day. Just reduce your attention to the news.

8. I cannot think of anything that is more stressful or futile than trying to change another person. The person will change when they want to, and you don't have to stress yourself by trying to get them change.

9. Studies have shown that people who have any pastimes, hobbies, and the like that they engage with frequently or every day demonstrate less stress and a greater sense of well-being. Also see # 3 above as these could also be used as distractions.

10. If you tend to overly indulge, such as in eating, drinking, or gambling, you are probably adding to your stress with guilt, if nothing else. You are not doing anything that is helpful for you when you overly indulge even in good things, such as exercise.

11. Do you overcommit your time and effort, that is, you take on too much? Some people who overcommit themselves also have an unrealistic expectation that they will also do everything perfectly or something similar. They take on too much and then are stressed when they find that they will not be able to do everything to their satisfaction. Worse is that they then displace some of their stress on their loved one.

Any of these can add to your stress. Even if you engage in a few of these, think of how you may feel better if you could just let them go.

11 Tips for Jump-starting Your Creativity

It is very easy to get caught up in our everyday tasks and demands, which make it difficult to be creative. However, there are some simple things you can do that could provide more incentive to do what you consider to be creative, whether that be writing, collaging, dancing, singing, cooking, working in the garden, or decorating—there are numerous ways to be creative. The challenge is to try and do something toward a creative product each day. The product does not have to be finished in a day; you just have to work on it daily or almost daily.

1. Make a list of what you think of as creativity for you such as cooking, drawing, collage, movement, or writing. Next, make a list of any materials you need to get started and locate these. Start small and modest. For example, if you want to make a collage, get an ATC (Artist Trading Card, which is a card the size of a playing card 23/4" × 3"), a magazine with images, a set of crayons or felt markers or colored pencils, scissors, scrap paper, and glue or glue sticks. This would be a small collage and could be inspiring and encouraging.

2. Begin the creative project; think, move, make a mark on paper, get spices for a new recipe, or anything related to your project.

3. Do something on your project every day, even if you just review your progress, or think about your next step. Keep it in the forefront of your thoughts.

4. Start a journal of ideas for creative projects. Sometimes you may just want to jot down your ideas for creative projects before embarking on one. Of several, pick one and then get on with it.

5. Learn a new technique connected with your creative project. Let's suppose that cooking is creative for you: what new techniques are there out in the

world that you could learn? You could search for a new technique on the internet, in a new book, or take a class. Try one new technique and see what happens.

6. Record what you do on your project and how you feel during the process. Do so in a journal, diary, calendar, or planning datebook. Or, make one of these your new project.

7. Teach someone else how to do what you are doing on your project. There could be someone who wants to learn how to do what you do, are intrigued by your product, or just want to hang out. Either way, both of you win.

8. Repurpose something, for example, a found object, something you possess, yesterday's newspaper. Use it for something other than its original intended purpose or in your creative project. For example, I use old newspapers a lot as backgrounds for collages and journal pages.

9. Try a new and different creative medium unlike your usual one; for example, if you write, try dance; if you sing, try drawing. I write, so when I want a change, I try to draw. You do not have to be good at the new and different medium; just the change can be enriching for you.

10. Take a class or workshop or view a DVD on a creative project. Learning from others is very helpful and can inspire and energize you.

11. Try an adult coloring book. These are supposed to be stress reducing, and the creative part comes with your color choices and the medium—pencils, crayons, ink, paint, gel, and so on.

After reading one or two of these, you can probably think of some better ideas for jump-starting your creative endeavors.

Index

About the Author

Nina W. Brown, EdD, is professor and eminent scholar of counseling at Old Dominion University in Norfolk, Virginia. She earned her doctorate at the College of William & Mary, and specializes in writings and studies on narcissism and group therapy. She is the author of 35 books, including several published also in Chinese, Polish, Turkish, German, and Korean. Her books include *Children of the Self-absorbed* (2008, 2015); *Loving the Self-absorbed* (2003); *Facilitating Challenging Groups* (2014); *Creative Activities for Group Therapy* (2013); *Uptight and In Your Face: Coping with an Anxious Boss, Parent, Spouse or Lover* (Praeger, 2013); *Dead-End Lovers: How to Avoid Them and Find True Intimacy* (Praeger, 2008); and *Coping with Infuriating, Mean, Critical People: The Destructive Narcissistic Pattern* (Praeger, 2006), plus eight additional books on group therapy. Brown is past president of the Society of Group Psychology and Group Psychotherapy (APA Division 49) and past secretary of the American Group Psychotherapy Association.